# Cardiac Home Exercise Guide & Workbook

## Plus

## Exercise Benefits & Precautions

## Lost Temple Fitness & Rehab

Karen Cutler: LPTA, ACE Certified Personal Trainer,
Medical, Cancer, Arthritis & Therapeutic Exercise Specialist

It is advised that you always check with your medical doctor or physical therapist before starting an exercise program or change in diet.

### Websites

LostTempleFitness.com

LostTempleFitnessCancer.com

LostTempleNutrition.com

LostTemplePets.com

LostTempleArt.com

# Introduction

It has been proven that exercise and nutrition are two of the main factors that you can control for a healthy lifestyle. Many people do not know how to start or progress an exercise program. There are hundreds of pictures for beginner, intermediate and advanced exercise programs, as well as a list of equipment that you can use in the home. This also includes worksheets to help you track your exercises and progress.

The cardiac section includes information on cardiac disease and stroke, including exercises that should be done for each health condition, as well as precautions and contraindications. Some of these diseases include, but not limited to, cardiomyopathy, atrial fibrillation and heart attack. This also includes precautions with pacemakers and defibrillators.

**This book is for:**

- Those with a history of heart disease, stroke or attending cardiac rehab to be used in conjunction with the physician or other health care provider and/or physical therapist recommendations.
- The beginner who has never exercised before.
- The individual that has mastered the basics but wants to know how to advance to the next level.
- Pre/post rehab individuals who would like to advance or want a list of exercise programs to follow.
- The personal trainer, physical therapist, or other coaches who would like their client to have a list of exercises that can be progressed or know more about precautions with clients or patients with cardiac disease.

**This book is not for or may need modification:**

- Chronic or acute disorders/injury's that is not being followed by a health care professional. This book can be used in conjunction with a rehab program.
- If you are over 40 and have never exercised before, it is advised that a physician clears you first.
- Undiagnosed pain.
- The person that does not feel they can safely modify their individual program, although can be used in conjunction with rehab or coaches/personal trainers.
- People with the following issues that have been cleared by an MD for an exercise program or in conjunction with rehab. These issues will be addressed in future volumes: Cancer, Diabetes, Respiratory disease and Arthritis.

**What is covered in this book?**

- Coronary Artery Disease
  - Stroke
  - Physical Activity and Heart
  - Exercise Response to Cardiac Medications
  - Cardiac disease or symptoms and possible exercise precautions
  - Hypertension / Hypotension
  - Cholesterol
  - Heart-healthy eating (NIH) Foods to Eat and Nutrients to Limit / DASH Diet

- Home Exercise Programs – pictures and explanations
  - Myofascial release
  - Flexibility – Stretching
  - Core Stability
  - Balance with progression to Standing Strengthening exercises
  - Strengthening
    - Lower extremity - Lying and Seated
    - Upper extremity
- Benefits and Factors to consider before starting an exercise program
- Vital signs and how to monitor exercise intensity
- Temperature – Heat and Cold
- Dehydration
- Anatomy
- Equipment needed for home exercise
- Warm up/cool down
- Duration, Frequency, Intensity and Primary Movement Patterns

## It is advised that you always check with your medical doctor or physical therapist before starting an exercise program or change in diet.

**INTRODUCTION**

# Cardiac
## *See Section for Specific TOC*

# HOME EXERCISE PROGRAM
## *See Section for Specific TOC*

# Cardiac Disease and Exercise

It is beneficial for people who have a history or are currently undergoing treatment for cardiac disease or stroke to engage in an exercise program. It has also been shown that a healthy diet and exercise program can decrease risk of cardiac issues before they happen, as well as help to decrease the risk of further events. Please read the second section of this book to see how exercise can help with endurance, balance, muscle strengthening and flexibility.

This book is for educational purposes and should not be substituted for the direction of a physician or other health care provider (*see Disclaimer*). Before starting an exercise program, especially if you have a history of cardiac disease or stroke, you should consult with a physician and/or physical/cardiac therapist. If directed to do so, you should start cardiac rehab and use this book with their recommendations.

Please read the 2<sup>nd</sup> section of this book to learn about precautions, even if you are a healthy individual and are reading this version to learn about preventing heart disease.

Most of the cardiac and stroke research is from the:
*CDC – Center for Disease Control and Prevention*
*NIH – National Heart, Blood and Lung Institute* (unless otherwise specified)
Please see **Cardiac References** for links.

***This book is not meant to substitute an exercise program prescribed by a health care professional but designed to accompany their recommendations.***
***Please consult with your physician before starting any exercise program.***

What is covered in this section?
- Coronary Artery Disease (CAD) aka Coronary Heart Disease (CHD)
  - Causes, Risk Factors and Medications
- Physical Activity and Your Heart
  - Levels of Intensity in Aerobic Activity
  - Types of Aerobic Activity
  - Other Types of Exercise; Risks
  - Benefits, Guidelines for Adults
  - Guidelines for Adults over 65 and Older
  - How to Make Physical Activity Part of your Daily Routine
- Exercise Response to Cardiac Medications:
  - Heart Rate (HR), Blood Pressure (BP) and Clinical Relevance
    - Beta Blockers, Nitrates, Calcium Channel Blockers, Digoxin, Diuretics, ACE inhibitors / ARB
- Cardiac Disease or Symptoms with Possible Exercise and Precaution Information
  - Angina, Arrhythmias, Atherosclerosis, Aortic Aneurysm, Atrial fibrillation, Pacemaker, Cardiomyopathy, Heart Attack, Heart Failure (CHF), Peripheral Arterial Disease (PAD)
- Hypertension/Hypotension
- Cholesterol
- Stroke aka Cerebrovascular accident (CVA)
  - Risk Factors, Signs and Symptoms, Complications, Treating Risk Factors
  - Hemorrhagic Stroke
  - Transient Ischemic Attack (TIA) aka Mini-Stroke
  - Exercise Programs by *National Stroke Association, Hope - A Stroke Recovery Guide* and *NIH – National Heart, Blood and Lung Institute*
- Heart-healthy eating (NIH) Foods to Eat and Nutrients to Limit
  - DASH Diet

# Coronary Heart Disease (CHD) aka Coronary Artery Disease (CAD)

Most of the cardiac and stroke research is from the:
*CDC – Center for Disease Control and Prevention*
*NIH – National Heart, Blood and Lung Institute* (unless otherwise specified)

## *Quick Summary* this Section

**What is CAD/CHD**
- CAD is caused by plaque buildup in the walls of the arteries that supply blood to the heart (called coronary arteries) and other parts of the body.

**Causes:**
- Coronary heart disease (CHD) starts when certain factors damage the inner layers of the coronary arteries.

**Major Risk Factors:**
- These include unhealthy cholesterol levels, high blood pressure, smoking, diabetes, insulin resistance, lack of exercise, unhealthy diet, age, obesity, metabolic disease, family history

**Emerging and other Risk Factors related to CAD:**
- These include high levels of C – reactive protein, inflammation, high levels of triglycerides, sleep apnea, stress, alcohol, preeclampsia (during pregnancy)

**Medications:**
- Sometimes lifestyle changes are not enough to control your blood cholesterol levels. For example, you may need statin medications to control or lower your cholesterol. By lowering your cholesterol level, you can decrease your chance of having a heart attack or stroke.

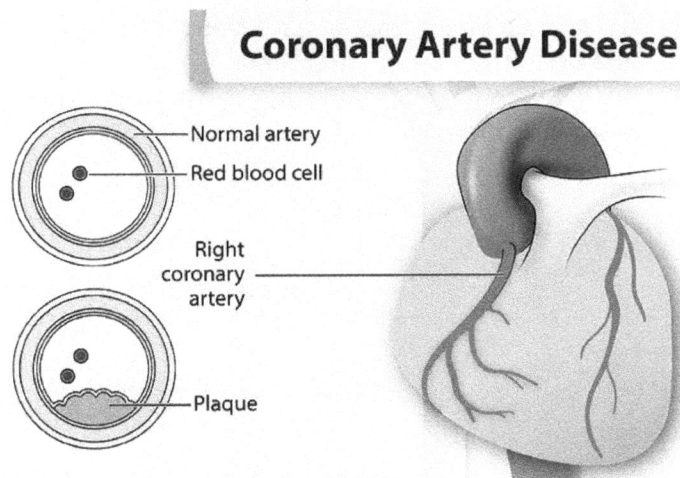

**Coronary Artery Disease**

Normal artery
Red blood cell
Right coronary artery
Plaque

**Picture - CDC**
*https://www.cdc.gov/heart-disease/about/coronary-artery-disease.html*

| | |
|---|---|
| **What is CAD/CHD**<br><br>*(CDC heart disease)*<br>and<br>*(NIH CHD)* | CAD is caused by plaque buildup in the walls of the arteries that supply blood to the heart (called coronary arteries) and other parts of the body.<br>• Plaque is made up of deposits of cholesterol and other substances in the artery. Plaque buildup causes the inside of the arteries to narrow over time, which could partially or totally block the blood flow.<br>    ○ This process is called **atherosclerosis**.<br>• Too much plaque buildup and narrowed artery walls can make it harder for blood to flow through your body.<br>    ○ When your heart muscle doesn't get enough blood, you may have chest pain or discomfort, called **angina**.<br>• **Angina** is the most common symptom of CAD.<br><br>Over time, CAD can weaken the heart muscle.<br>• This may lead to **heart failure,** a serious condition where the heart can't pump blood the way that it should.<br>• An irregular heartbeat, or **arrhythmia**, also can develop. |
| **Causes**<br><br>*(NIH CHD)* | Research suggests that coronary heart disease (CHD) starts when certain factors damage the inner layers of the coronary arteries.<br>**These factors include:**<br>• Smoking<br>• High levels of certain fats and cholesterol in the blood<br>• High blood pressure<br>• High levels of sugar in the blood due to insulin resistance or diabetes<br>• Blood vessel inflammation<br>• Plaque might begin to build up where the arteries are damaged. The buildup of plaquein the coronary arteries may start in childhood.<br><br>Over time, plaque can harden or rupture (break open).<br>• Hardened plaque narrows the coronary arteries and reduces the flow of oxygen-rich blood to the heart. This can cause *angina* (chest pain or discomfort).<br>• If the plaque ruptures, blood cell fragments called *platelets* stick to the site of the injury. They may clump together to form *blood clots.*<br>• *Blood clots* can further narrow the coronary arteries and worsen angina.<br>    ○ If a clot becomes large enough, it can mostly or completely block a coronary artery and cause a *heart attack*. |

| | |
|---|---|
| **Major Risk Factors** | **Major Risk Factors include:**<br>• Unhealthy blood *cholesterol* levels. This includes high LDL cholesterol (sometimes called "bad" cholesterol) and low HDL cholesterol (sometimes called "good" cholesterol).<br>• *High blood pressure.* Blood pressure is considered high if it stays at or above 140/90 mmHg over time. If you have diabetes or chronic kidney disease, high blood pressure is defined as 130/80 mmHg or higher. (The mmHg is millimeters of mercury—the units used to measure blood pressure.)<br>• *Smoking.* Smoking can damage and tighten blood vessels, lead to unhealthy cholesterol levels, and raise blood pressure. Smoking also can limit how much oxygen reaches the body's tissues.<br>• *Insulin resistance.* This condition occurs if the body can't use its own insulin properly. Insulin is a hormone that helps move blood sugar into cells where it's used for energy. Insulin resistance may lead to *diabetes.*<br>• *Diabetes.* With this disease, the body's blood sugar level is too high because the body doesn't make enough insulin or doesn't use its insulin properly.<br>• *Overweight or obesity.* The terms "overweight" and "obesity" refer to body weight that's greater than what is considered healthy for a certain height.<br>• *Metabolic syndrome.* Metabolic syndrome is the name for a group of risk factors that raises your risk for CHD and other health problems, such as diabetes and stroke.<br>• *Lack of physical activity.* Being physically inactive can worsen other risk factors for CHD, such as unhealthy blood cholesterol levels, high blood pressure, diabetes, and overweight or obesity.<br>• *Unhealthy diet.* An unhealthy diet can raise your risk for CHD. Foods that are high in saturated and trans fats, cholesterol, sodium, and sugar can worsen other risk factors for CHD.<br>• *Older age.* Genetic or lifestyle factors cause plaque to build up in your arteries as you age.<br>    o *In men,* the risk for coronary heart disease increases starting at age 45.<br>    o In *women,* the risk for coronary heart disease increases starting at age 55.<br>• *A family history of early coronary heart disease* is a risk factor for developing coronary heart disease, specifically if a father or brother is diagnosed before age 55, or a mother or sister is diagnosed before age 65.<br><br>Although older age and a family history of early heart disease are risk factors, it doesn't mean that you'll develop CHD if you have one or both.<br>• Controlling other risk factors often can lessen genetic influences and help prevent CHD, even in older adults. |

| | |
|---|---|
| **Emerging Risk Factors and Other Risks Related to Coronary Heart Disease** | **Researchers continue to study other possible risk factors for CHD.**<br>• *High levels of a protein called C-reactive protein (CRP)* in the blood may raise the risk of CHD and heart attack. High levels of CRP are a sign of inflammation in the body.<br>• *Inflammation* is the body's response to injury or infection. Damage to the arteries' inner walls may trigger inflammation and help plaque grow. Research is under way to find out whether reducing inflammation and lowering CRP levels also can reduce the risk of CHD and heart attack.<br>• *High levels of triglycerides* in the blood also may raise the risk of CHD, especially in women. Triglycerides are a type of fat.<br><br>**Other conditions and factors also may contribute to CHD, including:**<br>• *Sleep apnea.* Sleep apnea is a common disorder in which you have one or more pauses in breathing or shallow breaths while you sleep. Untreated sleep apnea can increase your risk for high blood pressure, diabetes, and even a heart attack or stroke.<br>• *Stress.* Research shows that the most commonly reported "trigger" for a heart attack is an emotionally upsetting event, especially one involving anger.<br>• *Alcohol.* Heavy drinking can damage the heart muscle and worsen other CHD risk factors. Men should have no more than two drinks containing alcohol a day. Women should have no more than one drink containing alcohol a day.<br>• *Preeclampsia.* This condition can occur during pregnancy. The two main signs of preeclampsia are a rise in blood pressure and excess protein in the urine. Preeclampsia is linked to an increased lifetime risk of heart disease, including CHD, heart attack, heart failure, and high blood pressure. |
| **Medications**<br><br>*See Exercise Response to Cardiac Medications* | Sometimes lifestyle changes are not enough to control your blood cholesterol levels.<br>• For example, you may need statin medications to control or lower your cholesterol.<br>• By lowering your cholesterol level, you can decrease your chance of having a heart attack or stroke.<br>• Doctors may discuss beginning statin treatment with those who have an elevated risk for developing heart disease or having a stroke<br><br>Doctors usually prescribe statins for people who have:<br>• Coronary heart disease, peripheral artery disease, or had a prior stroke<br>• Diabetes<br>• High LDL cholesterol levels<br><br>Your doctor also may prescribe other medications to:<br>• Decrease your chance of having a heart attack or dying suddenly.<br>• Lower your blood pressure.<br>• Prevent blood clots, which can lead to heart attack or stroke.<br>• Prevent or delay the need for a procedure or surgery, such as percutaneous coronary intervention or coronary artery bypass grafting.<br>• Reduce your heart's workload and relieve CHD. |

# Physical Activity and Your Heart (NIH)

*Please read 2nd section in the book to learn about Physical Activity and Exercise*

*NIH – National Heart, Blood and Lung Institute (unless otherwise specified)*

## Quick Summary of Section

**What is Physical Activity?**

- Physical activity is any body movement that works your muscles and requires more energy than resting. Walking, running, dancing, swimming, yoga, and gardening are a few examples of physical activity.

**Aerobic Activity**

- Aerobic activity moves your large muscles, such as those in your arms and legs. Running, swimming, walking, bicycling, dancing, and jumping jacks are examples of aerobic activity.

**Levels of Intensity in Aerobic Activity**

- You can do aerobic activity with light, moderate, or vigorous intensity.

**Examples of Aerobic Activities**

- Pushing a cart, gardening, water aerobics, tennis, hockey, walking, jogging, running

**Other Types of Physical Activity**

- Muscle-strengthening, bone strengthening, and stretching

**Exercise Risks**

- Rarely, heart problems occur as a result of physical activity.
- Examples of these problems include arrhythmias, sudden cardiac arrest, and heart attack.
- These events generally happen to people who already have heart conditions.

**Exercise Benefits**

- Physical activity reduces coronary heart disease risk factors
- Strengthening heart and lung function

**Guidelines for Adults**

- Some physical activity is better than none. Inactive adults should gradually increase their level of activity. People gain health benefits from as little as 60 minutes of moderate- intensity aerobic activity per week.

**Guidelines for Adults (Aged 65 or Older)**

- Older adults should be physically active. Older adults who do any amount of physical activity gain some health benefits.

**Make Physical Activity Part of Your Daily Routine**

- Do activities that you enjoy and make them part of your daily routine.
- If you haven't been active for a while, start low and build slow.

**Exercise Response to Cardiac Medications**

- B-blockers, Nitrates, Calcium channel blockers, Digoxin, Diuretics, ACE inhibitors

| | |
|---|---|
| **What is Physical Activity**<br><br>*(NIH – National Institutes of Health)* | Physical activity is any body movement that works your muscles and requires more energy than resting. Walking, running, dancing, swimming, yoga, and gardening are a few examples of physical activity.<br><ul><li>Exercise is a type of physical activity that's planned and structured. Lifting weights, taking anaerobics class, and playing on a sports team are examples of exercise.</li><li>Physical activity is good for many parts of your body.</li><li>A heart-healthy lifestyle also involves following a heart-healthy eating, aiming for a healthy weight, managing stress, and quitting smoking. (NIH)</li></ul> |
| **Aerobic Activity** | Aerobic activity moves your large muscles, such as those in your arms and legs.<br><ul><li>Running, swimming, walking, bicycling, dancing, and jumping jacks are examples of aerobic activity. Aerobic activity also is called endurance activity.</li><li>Aerobic activity makes your heart beat faster than usual. You also breathe harder during this type of activity.</li><li>Over time, regular aerobic activity makes your heart and lungs stronger and able to work better.</li></ul> |
| **Levels of Intensity in Aerobic Activity**<br><br>*(NIH & Harvard Medical Publishing)* | You can do aerobic activity with light, moderate, or vigorous intensity. Moderate- and vigorous-intensity aerobic activities are better for your heart than light-intensity activities. However, even light-intensity activities are better than no activity at all.<br><ul><li>The level of intensity depends on how hard you must work to do the activity. To do the same activity, people who are less fit usually must work harder than people who are fitter.</li><li>So, for example, what is light-intensity activity for one person may be moderate-intensity for another.</li></ul><br>**LIGHT- AND MODERATE-INTENSITY ACTIVITIES**<br>Light-intensity activities are common daily activities that do not require much effort<br><ul><li>Moderate-intensity activities make your heart, lungs, and muscles work harder than light-intensity activities do.</li><li>On a scale of 0 to 10, moderate-intensity activity is a 5 or 6 and produces noticeable increases in breathing and heart rate.</li><li>A person doing moderate-intensity activity can talk but not sing.</li></ul><br>**VIGOROUS-INTENSITY ACTIVITIES**<br>Vigorous-intensity activities make your heart, lungs, and muscles work hard. |

| **Example of Walking Intensity** *(Harvard Medical Publishing)* | | | |
|---|---|---|---|
| *Type of walking* | *Pace* | *How it feels* | *Intensity* |
| *Easy* | Leisurely stroll | Light effort, breathing easily. You can sing | Light |
| *Moderate* | Purposeful, like you havesome place to get to | Some effort, breathing morenoticeable. You can talk in full sentences | Light to moderate |
| *Brisk* | In a bit of a hurry | Moderate effort, breathing harder. You can talk in full sentences, but need to take more breaths | Moderate |
| *Fast* | Late for an appointment | Hard effort, slightly breathless. You can talk in phrases | Moderate to vigorous |

| | |
|---|---|
| **Examples of Aerobic Activities** | Below are examples of aerobic activities. Depending on your level of fitness, they can be light, moderate, or vigorous in intensity:<br>• Pushing a grocery cart around a store<br>• Gardening, such as digging or hoeing that causes your heart rate to go up<br>• Walking, hiking, jogging, running<br>• Water aerobics or swimming laps<br>• Bicycling, skateboarding, rollerblading, and jumping rope<br>• Ballroom dancing and aerobic dancing<br>• Tennis, soccer, hockey, and basketball |
| **Other Types of Physical Activity** | The other types of physical activity—*muscle-strengthening, bone strengthening,* **and** *stretching*—benefit your body in other ways.<br><br>• **Muscle-strengthening** activities improve the strength, power, and endurance of your muscles. Doing pushups and sit-ups, lifting weights, climbing stairs, and digging in the garden are examples of muscle-strengthening activities.<br><br>• With **bone-strengthening activities**, your feet, legs, or arms support your body's weight, and yourmuscles push against your bones. This helps make your bones strong. Running, walking, jumping rope, and lifting weights are examples of bone-strengthening activities.<br><br>• **Muscle-strengthening and bone-strengthening activities** also can be aerobic, depending on whether they make your heart and lungs work harder than usual. For example, running is both anaerobic activity and a bone-strengthening activity.<br><br>• **Stretching** helps improve your flexibility and your ability to fully move your joints. Touching your toes, doing side stretches, and doing yoga exercises are examples of stretching. |
| **Exercise Risks** | In general, the benefits of regular physical activity far outweigh risks to the heart and lungs.<br>• Rarely, heart problems occur as a result of physical activity. Examples of these problems include arrhythmias, sudden cardiac arrest, and heart attack. These events generally happen to people who already have heart conditions.<br>• The risk of heart problems due to physical activity is higher for youth and young adults who have congenital heart problems. The term *"congenital"* means the heart problem has been present since birth.<br>   o *Congenital heart problems* include hypertrophic cardiomyopathy, congenital heart defects, and myocarditis. People who have these conditions should ask their doctors what types of physical activity are safe for them.<br>• For middle-aged and older adults, the risk of heart problems due to physical activity is related to *coronary heart disease (CHD)*.<br>   o People who have CHD are more likely to have aheart attack when they are exercising vigorously than when they are not.<br>• The risk of heart problems due to physical activity is related to your fitness level and the intensity of the activity you are doing.<br>   o For example, someone who is not physically fit is at higher risk for a heart attack during vigorous activity than a person who is physically fit.<br>• **If you have a heart problem or chronic (ongoing) disease—such as heart disease, diabetes, or high blood pressure—ask your doctor what types of physical activity are safe for you.**<br>   o ***You also should talk with your doctor about safe physical activities if you have symptoms such as chest pain or dizziness.*** |

| | |
|---|---|
| **Exercise Benefits** | <ul><li>Physical activity strengthens your heart and improves lung function. When done regularly, moderate- and vigorous-intensity physical activity strengthens your heart muscle.<ul><li>This improves your heart's ability to pump blood to your lungs and throughout your body. As a result, more blood flows to your muscles, and oxygen levels in your blood rise.</li></ul></li><li>Capillaries, your body's tiny blood vessels, also widen. This allows them to deliver more oxygen to your body and carry away waste products.</li><li>Physical activity reduces coronary heart disease risk factors. When done regularly, moderate- and vigorous-intensity aerobic activity can lower your risk for CHD.<ul><li>Plaque narrows the arteries and reduces blood flow to your heart muscle. Eventually, an area of plaque can rupture (break open).</li><li>This causes a blood clot to form on the surface of the plaque. If the clot becomes large enough, it can mostly or completely block blood flow through a coronary artery.</li><li>Blocked blood flow to the heart muscle causes a heart attack.</li></ul></li></ul><br>Certain traits, conditions, or habits may raise your risk for CHD.<br>Physical activity can help control some of these risk factors because it:<ul><li>Can lower blood pressure and triglyceride.<ul><li>Triglycerides are a type of fat in the blood.</li></ul></li><li>Can raise HDL cholesterol levels.<ul><li>HDL sometimes is called "good" cholesterol.</li></ul></li><li>Helps your body manage blood sugar and insulin levels, which lowers your risk for type 2 diabetes.</li><li>Reduces levels of C-reactive protein (CRP) in your body.<ul><li>This protein is a sign of inflammation. High levels of CRP may suggest an increased risk for CHD.</li></ul></li><li>Helps reduce overweight and obesity when combined with a reduced-calorie diet.<ul><li>Physical activity also helps you maintain a healthy weight over time once you have lost weight.</li></ul></li><li>May help you quit smoking.<ul><li>Smoking is a major risk factor for CHD.</li></ul></li><li>Inactive people are more likely to develop CHD than people who are physically active.<ul><li>Studies suggest that inactivity is a major risk factor for CHD, just like high blood pressure, high blood cholesterol, and smoking.</li></ul></li></ul><br>Physical Activity Reduces Heart Attack Risk<ul><li>For people who have CHD, aerobic activity performed regularly helps the heart work better.<ul><li>It also may reduce the risk of a second heart attack in people who already have had heart attacks.</li></ul></li><li>***Vigorous aerobic activity may not be safe for people who have CHD.***<ul><li>*Ask your doctor what types of activity are safe for you.*</li></ul></li></ul> |

| | |
|---|---|
| **Guidelines for Adults** | **Guidelines**<br>• Some physical activity is better than none.<br>  ○ Inactive adults should gradually increase their level of activity.<br>  ○ People gain health benefits from as little as 60 minutes of moderate-intensity aerobic activity per week.<br>• For major health benefits, do at least 150 minutes (2 hours and 30 minutes) of moderate-intensity aerobic activity or 75 minutes (1 hour and 15 minutes) of vigorous-intensity aerobic activity each week.<br>  ○ Another option is to do a combination of both.<br>  ○ A general rule is that 2 minutes of moderate-intensity activity counts the same as 1 minute of vigorous- intensity activity.<br>• For even more health benefits, do 300 minutes (5 hours) of moderate-intensity aerobic activity or 150 minutes (2 hours and 30 minutes) of vigorous-intensity activity each week(or a combination of both).<br>  ○ The more active you are, the more you will benefit.<br>• When doing aerobic activity, do it for at least 10 minutes at a time.<br>  ○ Spread the activity throughout the week.<br>  ○ Muscle-strengthening activities that are moderate or vigorous intensity should be included 2 or more days a week.<br>  ○ These activities should work all ofthe major muscle groups (legs, hips, back, chest, abdomen, shoulders, and arms).<br>  ○ Examples include lifting weights, working with resistance bands, and doing sit-ups and pushups, yoga, and heavy gardening. |
| **Guidelines for Adults Aged 65 or Older** | **The guidelines advise that:**<br>• Older adults should be physically active.<br>  ○ Older adults who do any amount of physical activity gain some health benefits.<br>  ○ If inactive, older adults should gradually increase their activity levels and avoid vigorous activity at first.<br>• Older adults should follow the guidelines for adults, if possible.<br>  ○ Do a variety of activities,including walking.<br>  ○ Walking has been shown to provide health benefits and a low risk of injury.<br>• If you cannot do 150 minutes (2 hours and 30 minutes) of activity each week, be as physically active as your abilities and condition allow.<br>• You should do balance exercises if you are at risk for falls. *(See Balance)*<br><br>*If you have a chronic (ongoing) condition—such as heart disease, lung disease, or diabetes—ask your doctor what types and amounts of activity are safe for you.* |

| | |
|---|---|
| **Make Physical Activity Part of Your Daily Routine** | **Do activities that you enjoy and make them part of your daily routine.**<br>• If you have not been active for a while, start low and build slow.<br>• Many people like to start with walking and slowly increase their time and distance.<br>• You also can take other steps to make physical activity part of your routine.<br><br>**PERSONALIZE THE BENEFITS**<br>• People value different things. Some people may highly value the health benefits from physical activity. Others want to be active because they enjoy recreational activities, or they want to look better or sleep better.<br>• Some people want to be active because it helps them lose weight or it gives them a chance to spend time with friends.<br>• Identify which physical activity benefits you value. This will help you personalize the benefits of physical activity.<br><br>**BE ACTIVE WITH FRIENDS AND FAMILY**<br>• Friends and family can help you stay active.<br>　o For example, go for a hike with a friend, take dancing lessons with your spouse or play ball with your child.<br><br>**MAKE EVERYDAY ACTIVITIES MORE ACTIVE**<br>• You can make your daily routine more active.<br>　o For example, take the stairs instead of the elevator. Instead of sending e-mails, walk down the hall to a coworker's office. Rake the leaves instead of using a leaf blower.<br><br>**REWARD YOURSELF WITH TIME FOR PHYSICAL ACTIVITY**<br>• Sometimes, going for a bike ride or a long walk relieves stress after a long day.<br>• Think of physical activity as a special time to refresh your body and mind.<br><br>**KEEP TRACK OF YOUR PROGRESS**<br>• Consider keeping a log of your activity. A log can help you track your progress.<br>• Many people like to wear a pedometer (a small device that counts your steps) to track how much they walk every day.<br>• These tools can help you set goals and stay motivated.<br><br>**BE ACTIVE AND SAFE**<br>• Be active on a regular basis to raise your fitness level.<br>• Do activities that fit your health goals and fitness level.<br>　o Start low and slowly increase your activity level over time.<br>　o As your fitness improves, you will be able to do physical activities for longer periods and with more intensity.<br>• Spread out your activity over the week and vary the types of activity you do.<br>• Use the right gear and equipment to protect yourself.<br>　o For example, use bicycle helmets, elbow and knee pads, and goggles.<br>• Be active in safe environments.<br>　o Pick well-lit and well-maintained places that are clearly separated from car traffic.<br>　o Follow safety rules and policies, such as always wearing a helmet when biking.<br>• Make sensible choices about when, where, and how to be active.<br>　o Consider weather conditions, such as how hot or cold it is, and change your plans as needed. |

## Exercise Response to Cardiac Medications *(portions adapted from Heart Online)*

| Medications | Heart Rate | Blood Pressure | Clinical Relevance to Exercise |
|---|---|---|---|
| **β-Blockers** Any of a group of drugs (as propranolol) that combine with and block the activity of a beta-receptor to decrease the heart rate and force of contractions and lower high blood pressure and that are used especially to treat hypertension, angina pectoris, and ventricular and supraventricular arrhythmias | ↓ at rest and with exercise | ↓ at rest and with exercise | • Monitor for symptoms of hypotension or bradycardia* <br>• Intensity monitoring reliant on HR should be avoided |
| **Nitrates** Used in the treatment of angina pectoris and as preservatives in meat products. Some individuals have sensitivity to nitrates and may suffer from headache, diarrhea, or urticaria after ingesting. | ↑ at rest <br><br> ↑ or no change with exercise | ↓ at rest <br><br> ↓ or no change with exercise | • For acute use, hypotension and reflex tachycardia are common. <br>• Monitor HRand BP. <br>• Exercise should be stopped. <br>• Monitor symptoms of hypotension, Tachycardia and Angina |
| **Calcium channel blockers** Any of a class of drugs (as *verapamil*) that prevent or slow the influx of calcium ions into smooth muscle cells especially of the heart and that are used especially to treat some forms of angina pectoris and some cardiac arrhythmias | No change at rest or with exercise (Dihydropyridines) <br><br> or <br><br> ↓ at rest and with exercise (Verapamil and Diltiazem) | ↓ at rest and with exercise | • Monitor for symptoms of hypotension (+/- bradycardia) <br>• Dihydropyridines (e.g. amlodipine, felodipine, lercanidipine, nifedipine) have greatest effect peripherally and therefore work to lower BP. Tachycardia may occur as an infrequent adverse effect <br>• Verapamil and diltiazem depress sinoatrial and atrioventricular node conduction as well as causing peripheral vasodilation, therefore affect both HR and BP <br>• Intensity monitoring reliant on HR should be avoided |
| **Digoxin** A cardiotonic steroid C41H64O14 obtained from a foxglove (Digitalis lanata) and used especially to treat atrial fibrillation | ↓ in patients with AF and possibly CHF | No change at rest or with exercise | • Monitor for signs of bradycardia |

| Medications | Heart Rate | Blood Pressure | Clinical Relevance to Exercise |
|---|---|---|---|
| **Diuretics**<br>An agent that increases the excretion of urine | No change at rest or with exercise | No change or ↓ at rest or with exercise | • Monitor for symptoms of hypotension and unexpected rapid weight changes<br>• Over diuresis or fluid loss through vomiting or diarrhea in the presence of diuretics may exacerbate hypotension |
| **ACE inhibitor and ARB**<br>Any of a group of antihypertensive drugs (such as captopril) that relax arteries and promote renal excretion of salt and water by inhibiting the activity of angiotensin converting enzyme | No change at rest or with exercise | ↓ at rest and exercise | • Monitor for symptoms of hypotension |

- Heart rate (HR) and blood pressure (BP) should be assessed prior to undertaking a supervised exercise program.
- Pre exercise values that differ significantly from the individual's norms may require modification of the exercise program or medical review prior to commencing.
- Recent medication changes or up-titration may require modifications to the exercise program.
- Monitor sitting and standing BP for those with suspected postural hypotension and avoid sudden postural changes or exercises that may exacerbate this in these patients

- *Blockers with mixed beta and alpha blocking activity (e.g. carvedilol) influence peripheral arterioles as well as reducing HR.*
- *Hypotension may be more significant than when using other -Blockers which primarily affect HR alone*
- *β -Blockers with intrinsic sympathomimetic activity (pindolol, oxprenolol) lower resting heart rate only slightly, and are not often used in the management of heart failure*

*Adapted from American College of Sports Medicine (2013). ACSM's Guidelines for Exercise Testing and Prescription, Ninth Edition. Lippincott, Williams & Wilkins and Australian Medicines Handbook 2014 (online). Adelaide: Australian Medicines Handbook Pty Ltd*

*Source*: Heart Online : Exercise response to cardiac medications   www.heartonline.org.au/resources   Reviewed 11/2014

# Cardiac Disease or Symptoms with Possible Exercise and/or Precautions
### NIH – National Heart, Blood and Lung Institute (unless otherwise specified)

## Quick Summary this Section

**Angina**
- A symptom of coronary artery disease. Chest pain or discomfort that occurs when the heart muscle is not getting enough blood

**Arrythmias**
- Irregular or unusually fast or slow heartbeats.

**Atherosclerosis**
- This occurs when plaque builds up in the arteries that supply blood to the heart (called coronary arteries).

**Aortic Aneurysm**
- An aortic aneurysm is a balloon-like bulge in the aorta, the large artery that carries blood from the heart through the chest and torso.

**Atrial Fibrillation (A - Fib)**
- A type of arrhythmia that can cause rapid, irregular beating of the heart's upper chambers.

**Cardiomyopathy**
- Occurs when the heart muscle becomes enlarged or stiff. This can lead to inadequate heart pumping (or weak heart pump) or other problems.

**Congestive Heart Failure (CHF)**
- Called congestive heart failure because of fluid buildup in the lungs, liver, gastrointestinal tract, and the arms and legs. Heart failure occurs when the heart can't pump enough blood to meet the body's needs.

**Heart Attack (Myocardial Infarction)**
- This happens when the flow of oxygen-rich blood to a section of heart muscle suddenly becomes blocked and the heart can't get oxygen. If blood flow isn't restored quickly, the section of heart muscle begins to die.

**Palpitations**
- You may feel palpitations in your chest, throat, or neck during activity or when sitting still or lying down.

**Peripheral Arterial Disease (PAD)**
- Occurs when the arteries that supply blood to the arms and legs (the periphery) become narrow or stiff. PAD usually results from atherosclerosis, the buildup of plaque and narrowing of the arteries.

**Pacemaker**
- A pacemaker is a small device that's placed in the chest or abdomen to help control abnormal heart rhythms. This device uses electrical pulses to prompt the heart to beat at a normal rate.

**Implantable Cardioverter Defibrillator (ICD)**
- An implantable cardioverter defibrillator (ICD) is a small device that your doctor can put into your chest to help regulate an irregular heart rhythm, or an arrhythmia.

**Hypertension and Hypotension**
- Hypotension is abnormally low blood pressure.
- Hypertension is abnormally high blood pressure.

**Cholesterol and Triglycerides**
- Cholesterol travels through the blood on proteins called "lipoproteins." Two types of lipoproteins carry cholesterol throughout the body.

| **Angina**<br><br>*CDC<br>and<br>MedScape: Specific<br>Exercise Precautions* | **A symptom of coronary artery disease.**<br>• Chest pain or discomfort that occurs when the heart muscle is not getting enough blood.<br>• Angina may feel like pressure or a squeezing pain in the chest.<br>• The pain also may occur in the shoulders, arms, neck, jaw, or back. It may feel like indigestion.<br><br>**There are two forms of angina—stable or unstable:**<br>• *Stable angina* happens during physical activity or under mental or emotional stress.<br>• *Unstable angina* is chest pain that occurs even while at rest, without apparent reason.<br>  ○ *This type of angina is a medical emergency.* |
|---|---|

## Unstable Angina

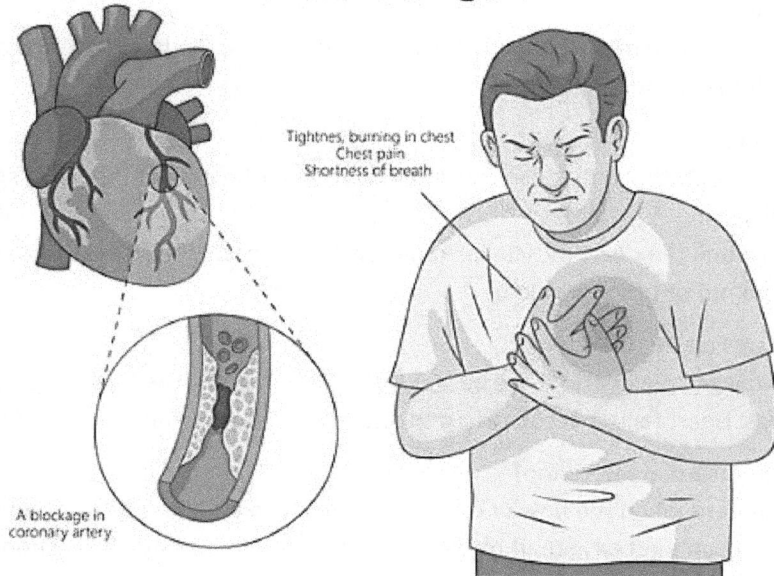

Tightnes, burning in chest
Chest pain
Shortness of breath

A blockage in coronary artery

**Exercise and/or Precautions**
- Stop exercising immediately if you experience angina.
- *Contact your physician if you experience chest pain, labored breathing, or extreme fatigue.*
- Upper-body exercises may precipitate angina more readily than lower-body exercises because of a higher press or response.
- An extended warm-up and cool-down may reduce the risk of angina or other cardiovascular complications following exercise.
- If nitroglycerin has been prescribed, always carry it with you, especially during exercise.
- Avoid extreme weather conditions.

| | Irregular or unusually fast or slow heartbeats. |
|---|---|
| ***Arrhythmias***<br><br>***Also see A-fib***<br><br>*CDC*<br>*and*<br>*Livestrong (Exercise)* | <ul><li>Arrhythmias can be serious.</li><li>One example is called ***ventricular fibrillation***.<ul><li>This type of arrhythmia causes an abnormal heart rhythm that leads to death unless treated right away with an electrical shock to the heart (called defibrillation).</li></ul></li><li>Other arrhythmias are less severe but can develop into more serious conditions, such as atrial fibrillation, which can cause a stroke.</li></ul>

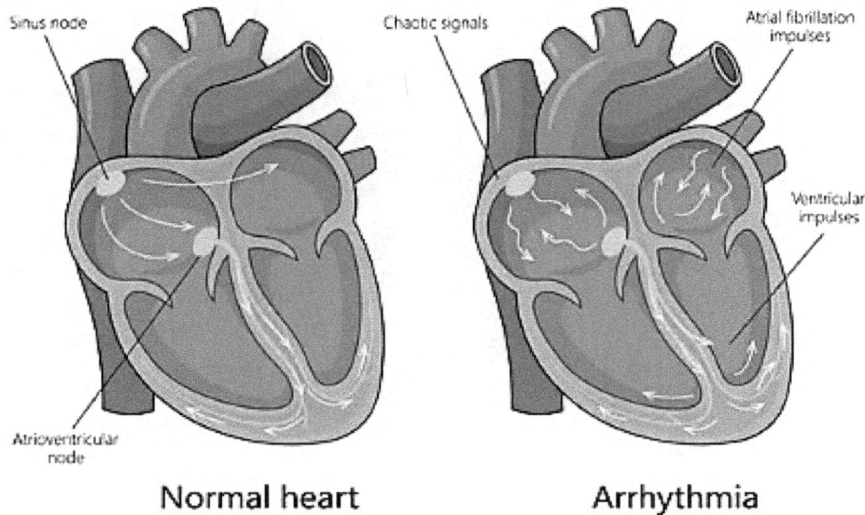

Cardiac Arrhythmia

Normal heart        Arrhythmia

**Exercise and /or Precautions** *(LiveStrong) – Also see **A-fib**.*
<ul><li>Do not overexert yourself during exercise; take breaks as needed, particularly if you feel your heart behaving abnormally.</li><li>Cool down by gradually reducing your activity after exercise to slowly return your heart rate back to a normal pace.<ul><li>For example, take a gentle 10-minute walk and stretch.</li></ul></li><li>If a certain type of exercise causes heart arrhythmias, discontinue it.</li><li>Avoid caffeinated beverages or foods and stop smoking.</li><li>Chronic heart arrhythmias may require an antiarrhythmic medication to help control episodes.</li></ul> |

| | |
|---|---|
| *Atherosclerosis*<br><br>*AKA*<br>**Arteriosclerosis**<br><br>**Hardening of the Arteries**<br><br>*CDC* and *NIH* | This occurs when plaque builds up in the arteries that supply blood to the heart (called *coronary arteries*).<br>• Plaque is made up of fat, cholesterol, calcium, and other substances found in the blood.<br>• Over time, plaque hardens and narrows your arteries. This limits the flow of oxygen-rich blood to your organs and other parts of your body.<br>• Atherosclerosis can lead to serious problems, including heart attack, stroke, or even death. |

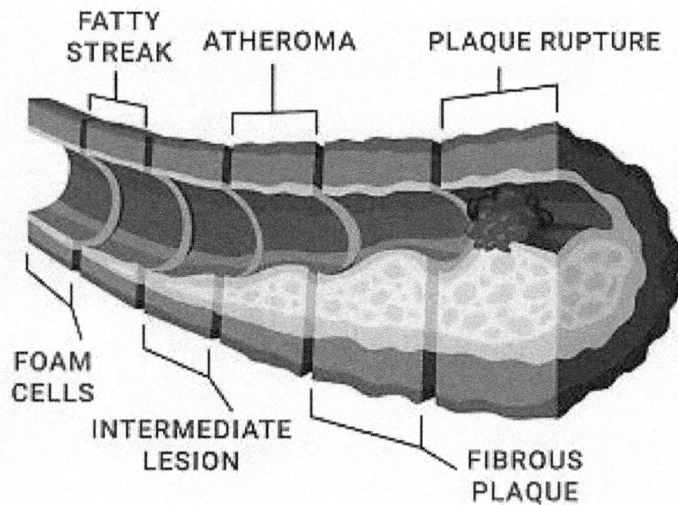

**Atherosclerosis-Related Diseases** *(See Particular Disease for More Information)*
- Atherosclerosis can affect any artery in the body, including arteries in the heart, brain, arms, legs, pelvis, and kidneys.
- Coronary Heart Disease / Coronary Artery Disease
- Peripheral Artery Disease
- Chronic Kidney Disease:
    - Can occur if plaque builds up in the renal arteries.
    - These arteries supply oxygen-rich blood to your kidneys.
    - Over time, chronic kidney disease causes a slow loss of kidney function.

## Aortic Aneurysm

*(CDC - Aortic Aneurysm, Livestrong and E-Pain assist)*

*Pic - CDC*

An aortic aneurysm is a balloon-like bulge in the aorta, the large artery that carries blood from the heart through the chest and torso.

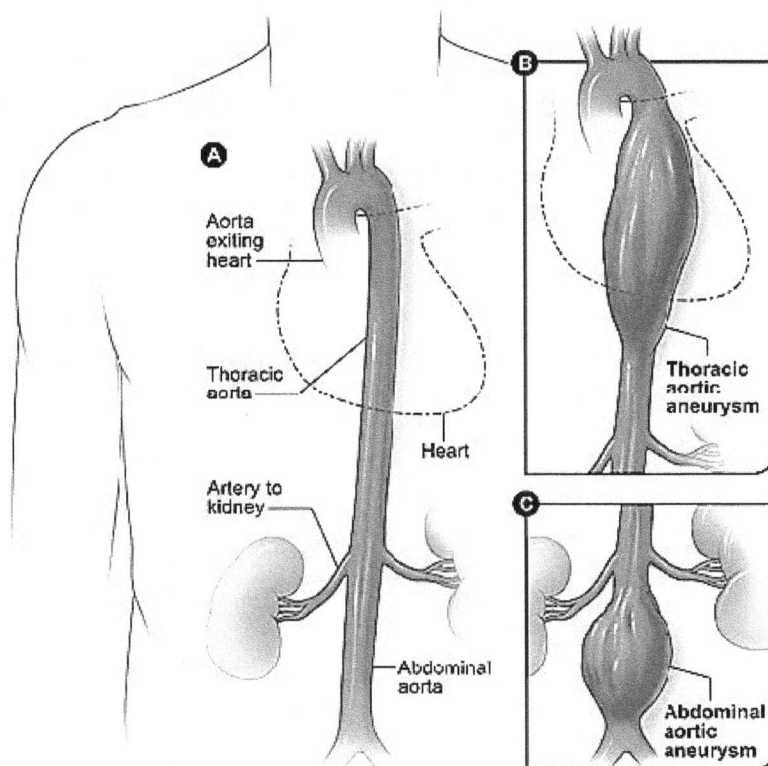

**Aortic aneurysms work in two ways:**
- *Dissections*
  - The force of blood pumping can split the layers of the artery wall, allowing blood toleak in between them.
  - This process is called a dissection.
- *Rupture*
  - The aneurysm can burst completely, causing bleeding inside the body.
- Dissections and ruptures are the cause of most deaths from aortic aneurysms.

**Thoracic Aortic Aneurysms.**
- A thoracic aortic aneurysm occurs in the chest.
- Men and women are equally likely to get thoracic aortic aneurysms, which become more common with increasing age.
- Thoracic aortic aneurysms are usually caused by high blood pressure or sudden injury.
- Sometimes people with inherited connective tissue disorders, such as Marfan syndrome and Ehlers-Danlos syndrome, get thoracic aortic aneurysms.

*Signs and symptoms of thoracic aortic aneurysm can include:*
- Sharp, sudden pain in the chest or upper back.
- Shortness of breath.
- Trouble breathing or swallowing

| | |
|---|---|
| *Aortic Aneurysm*<br><br>*Continued* | **Abdominal Aortic Aneurysms**<br>• An abdominal aortic aneurysm occurs below the chest.<br>• Abdominal aortic aneurysms happen more often than thoracic aortic aneurysms.<br>• Abdominal aortic aneurysms are more common in men and among people aged 65 years and older.<br>• Abdominal aortic aneurysms are less common among blacks compared with whites.<br>• Abdominal aortic aneurysms are usually caused by atherosclerosis (hardened arteries), but infection or injury can also cause them.<br><br>Abdominal aortic aneurysms often do not have any symptoms.<br>*If an individual does have symptoms, they can include:*<br>• Throbbing or deep pain in your back or side.<br>• Pain in the buttocks, groin, or legs.<br><br>Abdominal Aortic Aneurysm<br><br>Healthy abdominal aorta   Abdominal aorta with aneurysm<br><br>**Other Types of Aneurysms**<br>• Aneurysms can occur in other parts of your body.<br>• A ruptured aneurysm in the brain can cause a stroke.<br>• Peripheral aneurysms—those found in arteries other than the aorta—can occur in the neck, in the groin, or behind the knees.<br>   ○ These aneurysms are less likely to rupture or dissect than aortic aneurysms, but they can form blood clots. These clots can break away and block blood flow through the artery.<br><br>AORTIC ANEURYSMS |

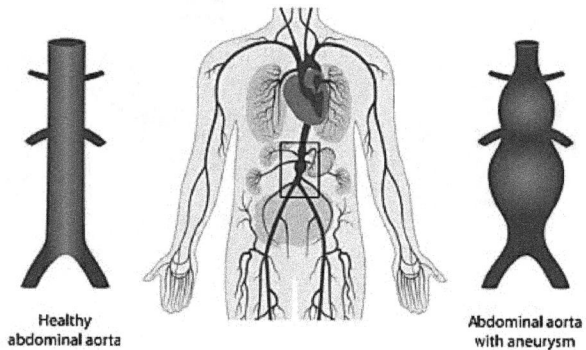

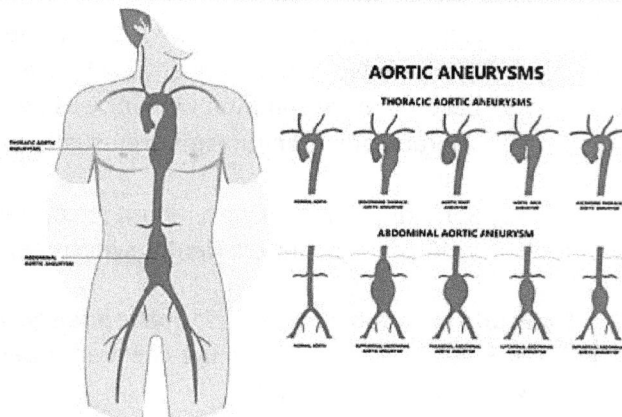

| **Aortic Aneurysm**<br><br>Continued<br><br>**Risk Factors**<br><br>**Treatments**<br><br>**Exercise and Precautions** | ***Risk Factors for Aortic Aneurysm***<br>Diseases that damage your heart and blood vessels also increase your risk for aortic aneurysm.<br>These diseases include:<br>• High blood pressure.<br>• High cholesterol.<br>• Atherosclerosis (hardened arteries).<br>• Smoking.<br>• Some inherited connective tissue disorders, such as Marfan syndrome and Ehlers-Danlos syndrome, can also increase your risk for aortic aneurysm. Your family may also have a history of aortic aneurysms that can increase your risk.<br>• Unhealthy behaviors can also increase your risk for aortic aneurysm, especially for people who have one of the diseases listed above.<br>    o Tobacco use is the most important behavior related to aortic aneurysm. People who have a history of smoking are 3 to 5 times more likely to develop an abdominal aortic aneurysm.<br><br>***Treating Aortic Aneurysm***<br>The two main treatments for aortic aneurysms are medicines and surgery.<br>• Medicines can lower blood pressure and reduce risk for an aortic aneurysm.<br>• Surgery can repair or replace the injured section of the aorta.<br><br>***Exercise and/or Precautions*** - *Exercise with AAA (LiveStrong)*<br>The root problem with AAAs is a weak vessel wall combined with high blood pressure.<br>• If you have been diagnosed with this condition, or there is a family history of aneurysms and dissections, it is important to perform *low intensity exercise* to avoid increasing your blood pressure to dangerous levels.<br>• A 2003 study in "JAMA" recommends patients with known aneurysms to exercise with *extreme caution*. The study recommends **limiting activities such as weightlifting because of the elevated risk of dissection**. *(LiveStrong)*<br><br>***What Are the Types of Exercise A Patient with Aortic Aneurysm Should Go for?***<br>*(E-Pain Assist)*.<br>The patient with aortic aneurysm should consult the doctor before starting with the exercise plan. In general, a patient with aortic aneurysm should keep the following points in mind while exercising:<br>• **Low Intensity**: A patient with aortic aneurysm may go for any form of low intensity exercise that does not carry a risk of the blood pressure shooting high suddenly.<br>• **Walking**: Brisk walking for 45 minutes to an hour is considered to be a good form of exercise for patients with aortic aneurysm. It keeps the body active and does not carry the risk of having high blood pressure.<br>• **Yoga**: The patient can go for yoga classes or aerobic exercises which are of characteristically low intensity to keep the body fit.<br>• ***Stay Away from Weightlifting***: A patient having aortic aneurysm should stay away from weightlifting because it tends to create a pressure on aorta which is dangerous.<br>    o ***It may cause rupturing of the aneurysm.*** |
|---|---|

| | |
|---|---|
| ***Atrial fibrillation***<br><br>*AKA*<br>***A-fib***<br><br><br>*CDC – A-fib,*<br>*HealthLine (HL),*<br>*Living with Atrial*<br>*Fibrillation*<br>*and*<br>*Everyday Health (EH)* | A type of arrhythmia that can cause rapid, irregular beating of the heart's upper chambers. Blood may pool and clot inside the heart, increasing the risk for heart attack and stroke.<br><br>**A-fib Symptoms:**<br>• Some people who have A-Fib do not know they have it and don't have any symptoms. Others may experience one or more of the following symptoms:<br>  ○ Irregular heartbeat<br>  ○ Heart palpitations (rapid, fluttering, or pounding)<br>  ○ Lightheadedness<br>  ○ Extreme fatigue<br>  ○ Shortness of breath<br>  ○ Chest pain<br><br>A-fib increases a person's risk for stroke by four to five times compared with stroke risk for people who do not have A-fib.<br>• Strokes caused by complications from A-fib tend to be more severe than strokes with other underlying causes.<br>• A-fib causes 15%–20% of ischemic strokes, which occur when blood flow to the brain is blocked by a clot or by fatty deposits called plaque in the blood vessel lining.<br><br>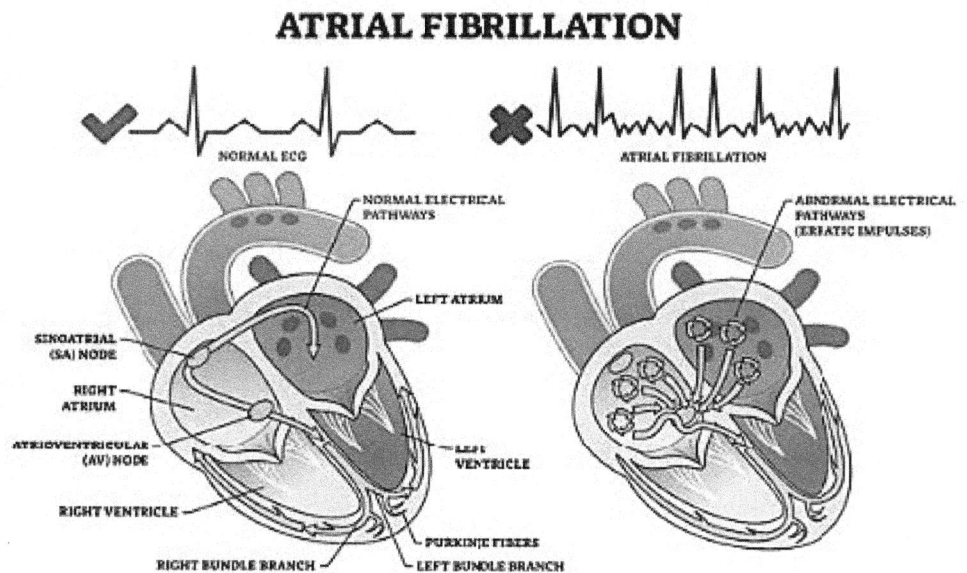<br><br>**Treatment for A-fib can include:**<br>• Medications to control the heart's rhythm and rate. Blood-thinning medication to prevent blood clots from forming and reduce stroke risk.<br>• Surgery. |

| | |
|---|---|
| *Atrial fibrillation*<br><br>*Continued*<br><br>**Exercise and Precautions** | ***Exercise and/or Precautions***<br><br>*Exercises to **avoid** with A-fib (HealthLine (HL) and Everyday Health (EH))*<br>• If you have not exercised in a while, you don't want to start with intense, high- impact exercise.<br>   o When you exercise with A-fib, you may want to start with short intervals of low-impact exercise.<br>   o Then you can gradually increase the length and intensity of your workouts. *(HL)*<br>• Try to avoid activities with a higher risk of causing injury, such as skiing or outdoor biking.<br>   o Many blood thinner medications used to treat A-fib may make you bleed more heavily when you're injured. *(HL)*<br>• If you plan to lift weights, talk to your doctor or a physical therapist about how much weight is safe for you to lift.<br>   o Lifting too much can put a lot of strain on your heart. *(HL)*<br>• Do not overheat. Some medications used to treat atrial fibrillation can lower your blood pressure, making you more sensitive to heat.<br>   o Protect yourself by taking frequent breaks, drinking water, and paying attention to how you feel.<br>   o If you feel dizzy or lightheaded during exercise, stop right away and cool off. *(EH)*<br>• Use an alternative method of heart rate monitoring. Because a-fib medications can slow down your pulse, checking your heart rate during exercise may not be effective, Stevens says.<br>   o Instead, for heart health and exercise safety, she recommends that you push yourself until your level of exertion is "somewhat hard" but you can still speak a full sentence without gasping.<br>   o "When people push to where they're working 'somewhat hard,' it usually corresponds to their target heartrate," she says. *(EH)*<br><br>***Beta Blockers and Exercise*** *(Living with Atrial Fibrillation)*<br>A-fib patients taking beta blockers must be aware that beta blockers naturally slow their heart rate.<br>• Your heart may not beat as fast even during exercise.<br>• As a result, checking or monitoring your heart rate while on these drugs may not be effective.<br>• A better guide in that situation is to listen to your body.<br>   o If you cannot speak a full sentence without gasping for air, you're pushing too hard.<br>   o You want to exercise to the point where you're tired and slightly winded, but can still talk without gasping for air. |

| | |
|---|---|
| ***Cardiomyopathy***<br><br>*CDC Cardiomyopathy and*<br>*Cardiomyopathy UK)* | Occurs when the heart muscle becomes enlarged or stiff. This can lead to inadequate heart pumping (or weak heart pump) or other problems.<br><br>• Cardiomyopathy has many causes, including family history of the disease, prior heart attacks, uncontrolled high blood pressure, and viral or bacterial infections.<br>• When cardiomyopathy occurs, the normal muscle in the heart can thicken, stiffen, thin out,or fill with substances the body produces that do not belong in the heart muscle.<br>    ○ As a result, the heart muscle's ability to pump blood is reduced, which can lead to irregular heartbeats, the backup of blood into the lungs or rest of the body, and heart failure.<br>• Cardiomyopathy can be acquired—developed because of another disease, condition, or factor—or inherited. The cause is not always known. |

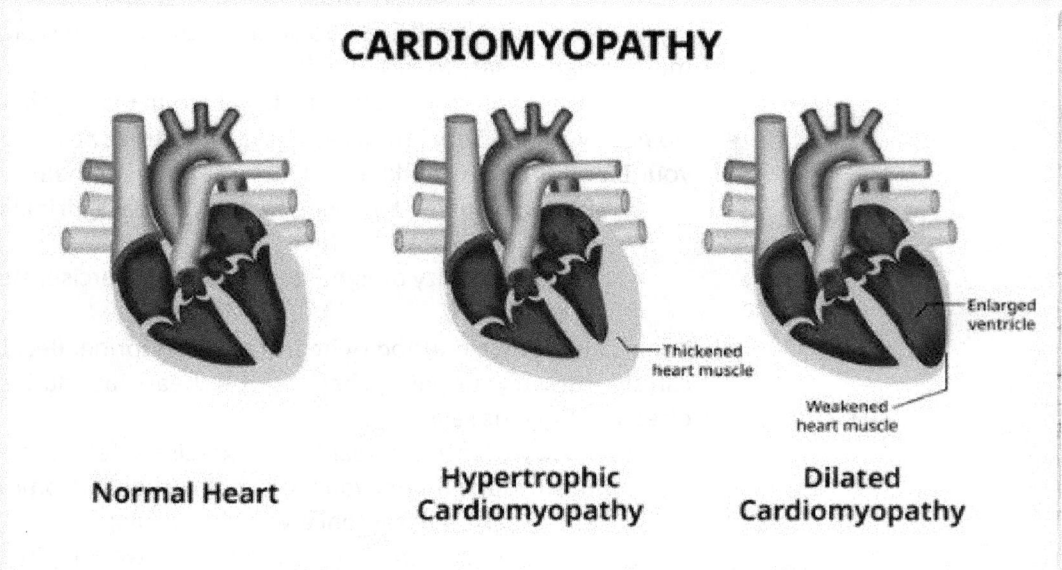

The main types of cardiomyopathies include the following:

• **Dilated**: where one of the pumping chambers (ventricles) of the heart is enlarged. This is more common in males and is the most common form of cardiomyopathy in children. It can occur at any age and may or may not be inherited.
• **Hypertrophic**: where the heart muscle is thickened. This often presents in childhood or early adulthood and can cause sudden death in adolescents and young adult athletes. It is often an inherited condition, and a person may not have any symptoms. If there is a family history of this, other family members can be tested and adjust their activities to reduce the risk of sudden death.
• **Arrhythmogenic**: where the disease causes irregular heartbeats or rhythms. This is often inherited and more common in males.
• **Restrictive**: where heart muscle is stiff or scarred, or both. It can occur with amyloidosis or hemochromatosis, and other conditions. This is the least common type.

Some people who have cardiomyopathy never have symptoms, while others may show signs as the disease progresses. These might include the following:

• Shortness of breath or trouble breathing.
• Fatigue.
• Swelling in the ankles and legs.
• Irregular heartbeat or palpitations.
• Syncope, the medical term for fainting or briefly passing out.

## Cardiomyopathy

*Continued*

*Pic/Chart - JACC Journal https://www.jacc.org/doi/10.1016/j.jacc.2022.07.013*

### Treatment and Prevention

- The goal of treatment is to slow down the disease, control symptoms, and prevent sudden death.
  - If you are diagnosed with cardiomyopathy, your doctor may tell you to change your diet and physical activity, reduce stress, avoid alcohol and other drugs, and take medicines.
  - Your doctor may also treat you for the conditions that led to cardiomyopathy, if they exist, or recommend surgery.
  - Treatment also depends on which type of cardiomyopathy you
- Genetic or inherited types of cardiomyopathies cannot be prevented but adopting or  following a healthier lifestyle can help control symptoms and complications.
- If you have an underlying disease or condition that can cause cardiomyopathy, early treatment of that condition can help prevent the disease from developing.

### Exercise and/or Precautions

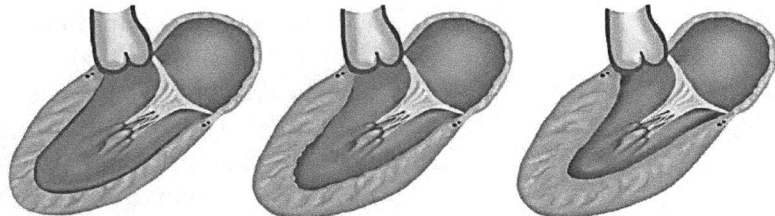

**CENTRAL ILLUSTRATION: Approach to Exercise Decision-Making in Hypertrophic Cardiomyopathy**

| Symptoms Past Medical History | Asymptomatic Good Functional Capacity | Symptoms Attributed to HCM With No Clear Association with Exercise | History of Cardiac Arrest or Unexplained Syncope*, Exercise-Induced Symptoms |
|---|---|---|---|
| HCM Risk-SCD Calculator | Low risk | Moderate risk | High risk |
| LVOT Gradient | No/mild LVOT gradient at rest or exercise (<30 mm Hg) + | Moderate LVOT gradient at rest or exercise (30-49 mm Hg) + | High LVOT gradient at rest or exercise (≥50 mm Hg) + |
| BP Response to Exercise | Normal + | Attenuated (<20 mm Hg increase in systolic BP) + | Systolic BP drop + |
| Exercise-Induced Arrhythmia | No arrhythmia ↓ When all applicable | Exercise-induced PVCs ↓ When ≥1 parameter applicable AND no parameter falls within the low-intensity column | Exercise-induced nonsustained or sustained ventricular tachycardia ↓ When ≥1 parameter applicable |
| Intensity of Exercise | High intensity | Moderate intensity | Low intensity |

Semsarian C, et al. J Am Coll Cardiol. 2022;80(13):1268-1283.

*JACC Journal https://www.jacc.org/doi/10.1016/j.jacc.2022.07.013*

| | |
|---|---|
| *Cardiomyopathy*<br><br>*Continued*<br><br>**Exercise and Precautions**<br><br>*Breathing Difficulties*<br><br>*Different Types*<br><br>*Exercise with ICD* | **Exercise and breathing difficulties.** *(Cardiomyopathy UK)*<br>How much your condition affects your ability to do physical activity is sometimes classified by the 'New York Heart Association classification of heart failure'. This looks at difficulty in breathing during different levels of activity for people with heart failure (where the heart is unable to meet the normal demands of the body).<br><br>• **Class I** (unaffected): no limitations to activities. Ordinary activity doesn't cause symptoms.<br>• **Class II** (mildly affected): some limitation in activity. Moderately strenuous activity (such as walking up several flights of stairs) causes some symptoms such as tiredness, palpitations, and breathlessness.<br>• **Class III** (moderately affected): more limited activity than class II. Symptoms happen at low levels of activity (such as walking on a flat surface).<br>• **Class IV** (severely affected): very limited activity as symptoms happen with all physical activity, and the person is breathless even when resting.<br><br>**Exercise and different types of cardiomyopathies**<br>• Intensive or competitive exercise is NOT recommended for anyone with cardiomyopathy.<br>• *Arrhythmic* cardiomyopathy (or arrhythmogenic right ventricular cardiomyopathy or ARVC) - some types of exercise make this condition worse and can increase arrhythmias and symptoms of heart failure in some people. Exercise for people with this condition needs to be considered carefully and specifically individualized, as it can be dangerous in people whose condition is unstable.<br>• *Dilated cardiomyopathy (DCM)* - for people who are on medication, with stable symptoms and who do not have heart failure or arrhythmias, exercise can be important. It can help to improve symptoms and is not likely to affect the underlying condition. How much exercise to do depends on the person's symptoms.<br>• *Hypertrophic cardiomyopathy (HCM)* - it is not clear whether it can increase the thickening of the heart, and in some people it can cause arrhythmias. If an arrhythmia is picked up during an exercise test during diagnosis, the person may be considered for an ICD (to control any future arrhythmias).<br><br>***Exercising with an ICD (implantable cardioverter defibrillator).***<br>Some people are concerned that a change in their heart rate due to exercise could cause their ICD to give them a shock. Generally, people with an ICD can exercise, and an ICD is no more likely to give a shock during exercise than at any other time.<br><br>• ICDs should give a shock when they detect abnormal, dangerous, heart rhythms (arrhythmias). These arrhythmias are usually faster (higher heart rate) than what happens during normal exercise. An exercise test may be helpful to program the ICD to check that it recognizes the person's normal heart rate and only gives a shock at the appropriate time.<br>• ICDs are made up of a generator (which generates the shock if it is needed), a battery (to power the device) and leads (wires that connect the ICD to the heart). For many people, after they have recovered from having it implanted, their ICD does not limit their physical movement.<br>    o However, for some over-stretching the arm and shoulder could affect the leads. This may limit their movement and affect what exercise is suitable. This is something that they can discuss with their doctor.<br>• For some people, doing regular exercise might help to reduce the risk of arrhythmias. For anyone with an ICD, it is a good idea to warm up before, and to cool down after exercise. This helps to ensure that their heart rate increases and decreases gradually. This also reduces the risk of arrhythmias. |

| | |
|---|---|
| ***Congestive Heart Failure (CHF)*** <br><br><br> *AKA* <br> **Heart Failure** <br><br> *CDC,* <br> *NIH– HeartFailure,* <br> *AUSmed (AU),* <br> and <br> *Doctor's Handbook* <br> *(DH)* | Often called congestive heart failure because of fluid buildup in the lungs, liver, gastrointestinal tract, and the arms and legs. <br> • Heart failure is a serious condition that occurs when the heart cannot pump enough blood to meet the body's needs. It does not mean that the heart has stopped but that muscle is too weak to pump enough blood. <br> • The majority of heart failure cases are chronic or long-term heart failures. <br> • The only cure for heart failure is a heart transplant. However, heart failure can be managed with medications or medical procedures. <br><br> Conditions that damage or overwork the heart muscle can cause heart failure. <br> • Over time, the heart weakens. It is not able to fill with and/or pump blood as well as it should. <br> • As the heart weakens, certain proteins and substances might be released into the blood. These substances have a toxic effect on the heart and blood flow, and they worsen heart failure. <br><br> 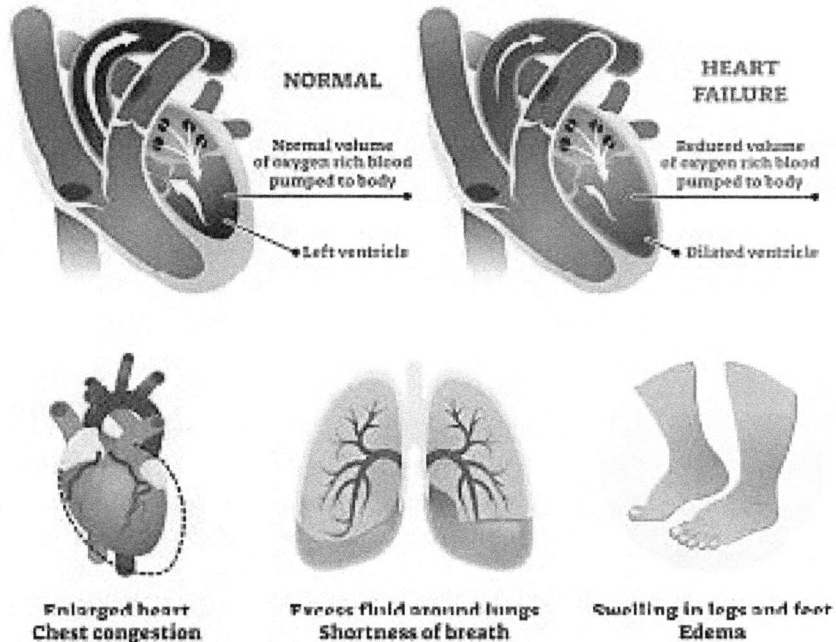 <br><br> **Causes of heart failure include:** <br> • Coronary heart disease <br> • Diabetes <br> • High blood pressure <br> • Other heart conditions or diseases <br>   o Arrhythmia. <br>   o Cardiomyopathy. <br>   o Congenital heart defects. Problems with the heart's structure are present at birth. <br>   o Heart valve disease. Occurs if one or more of your heart valves does not work properly, which can be present at birth or caused by infection, otherheart conditions, and age. |

| | |
|---|---|
| *Congestive Heart Failure (CHF)*<br><br>*Continued*<br><br>*Symptoms*<br><br>*Treatment*<br><br>*Exercise and Precautions* | **Common symptoms of heart failure include:**<br>• Shortness of breath during daily activities.<br>• Having trouble breathing when lying down.<br>• Weight gain with swelling in the feet, legs, ankles, or stomach.<br>• Generally feeling tired or weak.<br>   o All these symptoms are the result of fluid buildup in your body. When symptoms start, you may feel tired and short of breath after routine physical effort, like climbing stairs.<br>   o As your heart grows weaker, symptoms get worse. You may begin to feel tired and short of breath after getting dressed or walking across the room. Some people have shortness of breath while lying flat.<br>   o Fluid buildup from heart failure also causes weight gain, frequent urination, and a cough that is worse at night and when you're lying down.<br>      ❖ This cough may be a sign of acute pulmonary edema. This is a condition in which too much fluid builds up in your lungs. *The condition requires emergency treatment.*<br><br>**Treating Heart Failure**<br>• Early diagnosis and treatment can improve quality and length of life for people who have heart failure.<br>• Treatment usually involves taking medications, reducing sodium in the diet, and getting daily physical activity.<br>• People with heart failure also track their symptoms each day so that they can discuss these symptoms with their health care team.<br><br>**Exercise and/or Precautions** *(AUSmed (unless specified DH)*<br>• Specific contraindications to exercise in patients with CHF include new onset atrial fibrillation, obstructive valvular disease, especially aortic stenosis, or active myocarditis (either viral or autoimmune). *(DH)*<br>• CHF patients with ***diastolic and systolic dysfunction should*** refrain ***from swimming***. *(DH)*<br>• Recent studies show – if cardiac exercise is properly administered and supervised –a huge spectrum of patients with HF can safely participate, including patients with both systolic and diastolic dysfunction, atrial fibrillation, pacemakers, implantable cardioversion devices, and post-cardiac transplantation.<br>• Patients who are unstable or decompensated should not participate in exercise until stable; in fact, some programs will not permit patients to exercise until they have been *stable for 3 months or more*.<br>• No matter the official diagnoses, no HF patient is considered appropriate for exercise training until they are evaluated and assessed for current physical status, medical regime, and exercise tolerance.<br>• Patients should undergo an assessment with particular attention paid to signs or symptoms related to heart failure, such as the presence of new heart sounds, lung crackles, weight gain, or edema. |

*Congestive
Heart Failure*

Continued

*Signs and Symptoms*

*Risks*

### Chronic Heart Failure and Exercise Red Flags

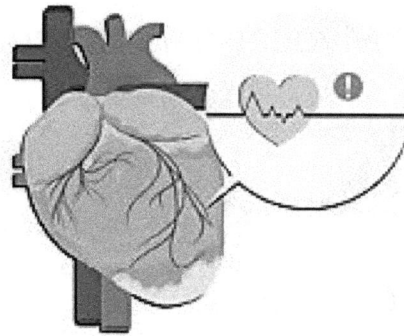

Symptoms of
# Heart Disease
## Heart Failure

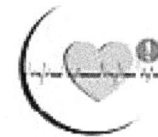

Rapid heartbeat

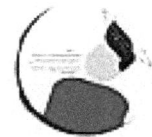

Fainting (Syncope)

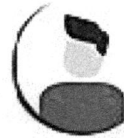

Chest pain

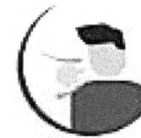

Shortness of breath

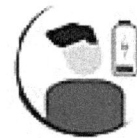

Fatigue

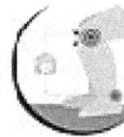

Edema

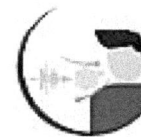

Wheezing

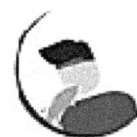

Nausea

### Signs and symptoms during exercise include:
- Hypotension (typically after exercise),
- Arrhythmias (both atrial and ventricular)
- A general worsening of CHF symptoms (dyspnea, swelling, etc.).
- Many patients with CHF already experience vacillating levels of symptoms from day to day; when this is the case, it is harder to determine if any decline in status is due to the exercise program or the disease itself.

### Unstable symptoms may include:
- Dyspnea: at rest/orthopnea (change from baseline), sudden onset of shortness of breath (SOB), worsening SOB, exertional dyspnea, gasping
- Arterial oxygen saturation (SaO2) less than 90%
- Coughing up pink/frothy sputum
- Dizziness or syncope
- Chest pain
- Systolic blood pressure (BP) less than 80 to 90mmHg and symptomatic
- Evidence of hypoperfusion (cyanosis, decreased level of consciousness, etc.)

### *Why is the CHF patient a special risk?*
- The body reacts differently to exertion and do not experience the normal physiological and compensatory responses that are commonly seen during an exercise session.
- Multiple medications including beta blockers, ACE inhibitors and diuretics, all of which dramatically alter how the heart responds to exercise stimuli.
- Pacemaker, implantable defibrillator or other device may alter the capacity to respond to exercise.
- Patients who have developed heart failure typically have a history of hypertension, coronary artery disease and/or diabetes. Each of these comorbidities brings its own special needs to the exercise table.

**Heart Attack**

*AKA*
***Myocardial infarction***

*CDC,*
*NIH*
*and*
*Cleveland Clinic*

Coronary artery disease (CAD) is the main cause of heart attack.
- A heart attack happens when the flow of oxygen-rich blood to a section of heart muscle suddenly becomes blocked and the heart cannot get oxygen.
- If blood flow is not restored quickly, the section of heart muscle begins to die.
- A less common cause is a severe spasm, or sudden contraction, of a coronary artery that can stop blood flow to the heart muscle.

## Myocardial infarction

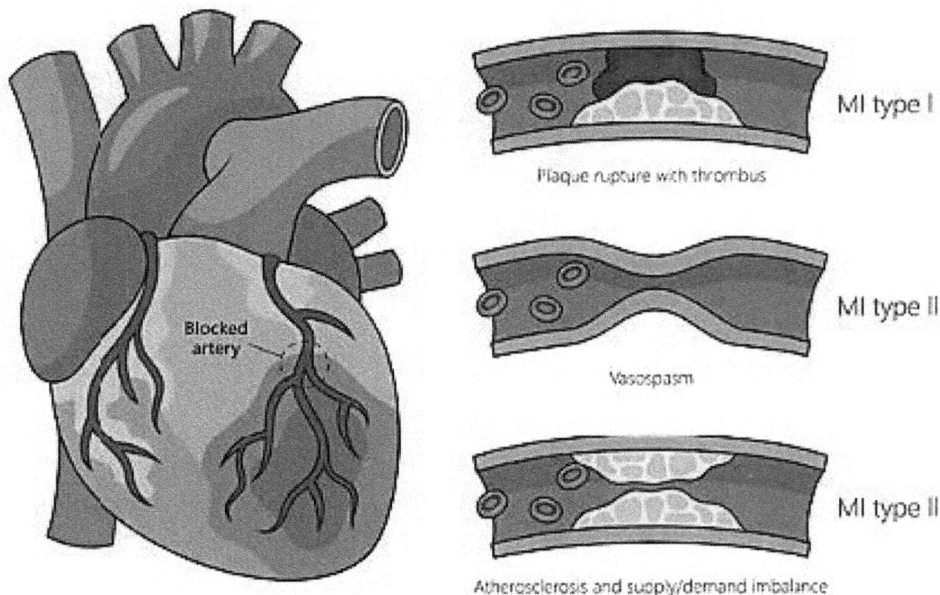

Blocked artery

MI type I
Plaque rupture with thrombus

MI type II
Vasospasm

MI type II
Atherosclerosis and supply/demand imbalance

Not all heart attacks begin with the sudden, crushing chest pain that often is shown on TV or in the movies. In one study, for example, one-third of the patients who had heart attacks had no chest pain. These patients were more likely to be older, female, or diabetic.
- The symptoms of a heart attack can vary from person to person. Some people can have few symptoms and are surprised to learn they have had a heart attack.
- If you have already had a heart attack, your symptoms may not be the same for another one.

It is important for you to know the most common symptoms of a heart attack and remember these facts:
- Heart attacks can start slowly and cause only mild pain or discomfort. Symptoms can be mild or more intense and sudden. Symptoms also may come and go over several hours.
- People who have high blood sugar (diabetes) may have no symptoms or very mild ones.
- The most common symptom, in both men and women, is chest pain or discomfort.
- Women are somewhat more likely to have shortness of breath, nausea and vomiting, unusual tiredness (sometimes for days), and pain in the back, shoulders, and jaw.
- Some people do not have symptoms at all. Heart attacks that occur without any symptoms or with very mild symptoms are called *silent heart attacks*.

| | |
|---|---|
| *Heart Attack*<br><br>*Continued*<br><br>*Pic CDC –*<br>*https://www.cdc.gov/hear*<br>*t-disease/about/heart-*<br>*attack.html*<br><br><br>*Symptoms*<br><br>*Lifestyle Changes* | **Most Common Symptoms:**<br>• ***Chest pain or discomfort***. Most heart attacks involve discomfort in the center or leftside of the chest. The discomfort usually lasts for more than a few minutes or goes away and comes back. It can feel like pressure, squeezing, fullness, or pain. It also can feel like heartburn or indigestion. The feeling can be mild or severe.<br>• ***Upper body discomfort.*** You may feel pain or discomfort in one or both arms, the back, shoulders, neck, jaw, or upper part of the stomach (above the belly button).<br>• ***Shortness of breath.*** This may be your only symptom, or it may occur before or along with chest pain or discomfort. It can occur when you are resting or doing a little bit of physical activity.<br>• ***The symptoms of angina can be similar to the symptoms of a heart attack***. Angina is chest pain that occurs in people who have coronary heart disease, usually when they are active. Angina pain usually lasts for only a few minutes and goes away with rest.<br>• Chest pain or discomfort that doesn't go away or changes from its usual pattern (for example, occurs more often or while you're resting) can be a sign of a heart attack.<br><br><br><br>**If you have had a heart attack**, your heart may be damaged. This could affect your heart's rhythm, pumping action, and blood circulation.<br>• You also may be at risk for another heart attack or conditions such as stroke, kidney disorders, and peripheral arterial disease (PAD).<br><br>**You can lower your chances** of having future health problems following a heart attack with these steps:<br>• Physical Activity<br>• Talk to your health care team about the things you do each day in your life and work.<br>• Your doctor may want you to limit work, travel, or sexual activity for sometime after a heart attack.<br><br>**Lifestyle Changes**<br>• Eating a healthier diet, increasing physical activity, quitting smoking, and managing stress—in addition to taking prescribed medications—can help improve your heart health and quality of life.<br>• Ask your health care team about attending a program called cardiac rehabilitation to help you make these lifestyle changes. |

| | |
|---|---|
| *Heart Attack*<br><br>*Continued*<br><br>*Cleveland Clinic*<br><br>***Exercise* and *Precautions*** | ***Exercise and/or Precautions*** *(Cleveland Clinic)*<br>After a heart attack it is important to begin a regular activity program to help reduce the chance of having additional heart problems.<br>• Your doctor will let you know when it is the right time to begin an exercise program. Most patients are given a prescription for Cardiac Rehabilitation.<br>• Patients who join cardiac rehabilitation programs have a faster and safer recovery and better outcomes after a heart attack. It is important to follow your cardiac rehabilitation team's instructions for activity.<br><br>Everyone recovers at a different pace. This may be related to your activity level before your heart attack or the amount of damage to your heart muscle. It may take many months to develop the optimal exercise program.<br>Here are some general guidelines from our cardiac rehabilitation staff to get started.<br>• Enroll in an outpatient cardiac rehab program to assist with developing the best exercise program and assisting with lifestyle changes such as heart healthy diet, quitting smoking, weight loss and stress management. Cardiac rehabilitation is covered by most insurance companies for patients after a heart attack.<br>• Returning to exercise after a heart attack or beginning a new exercise program can be challenging or anxiety provoking. Starting will small amounts and steadily building your program over time will help to set you up for success. A cardiac rehabilitation program will provide you with the support you need to get on a heart healthy path.<br>• Start slowly and gradually increase your walking pace over 3 minutes until the activity feels moderate (slightly increased breathing but should still be able to talk with someone). If you feel too short of breath, slow down your walking pace.<br>• Walk at a moderate pace for about 10 minutes the first time and each day try to add one or two minutes. By the end of a month, aim for walking 30 minutes most days of the week.<br>• Remember to cool down at the end of your exercise by gradually walking slower for the last 3 minutes of your exercise.<br>• If walking outside, walk with someone or in short distances close to home so you do not get too far away and have a hard time walking home.<br>• Choose an activity that you enjoy such as walking (outside or on a treadmill), stationary cycling, rowing, or water aerobics.<br>• ***Ask your doctor before lifting weights.***<br>• Exercise should be done regularly to gain the benefits; national guidelines suggest most days of the week if not every day.<br>• Try to exercise at the same time every day to establish a habit and to minimize any variables that may impact your exercise (timing of meals, medications, work schedule, etc.)<br>• If you notice any symptoms such as excessive shortness of breath, chest discomfort, palpitations that do not go away or increasing fatigue, stop your exercise and notify your doctor.<br>• After a heart attack many things may have changed including energy level and medications. These may affect your exercise tolerance; keep your exercise expectations day to day as you go through the healing process. |

## Palpitations

*NIH Palpitations*

You may feel palpitations in your chest, throat, or neck during activity or when you are sitting still or lying down.

- Strong emotions, physical activity, some medicines, caffeine, alcohol, nicotine, or illegal drugs may cause palpitations.
- Medical conditions such as thyroid disease, low blood sugar, anemia, and low blood pressure also may cause palpitations.
- Heart palpitations may be a sign or symptom of arrhythmia, an irregular heartbeat, or other heart conditions such as heart attack, heart failure, heart valve disease, or cardiomyopathy.

### Normal and Abnormal Heart Rate

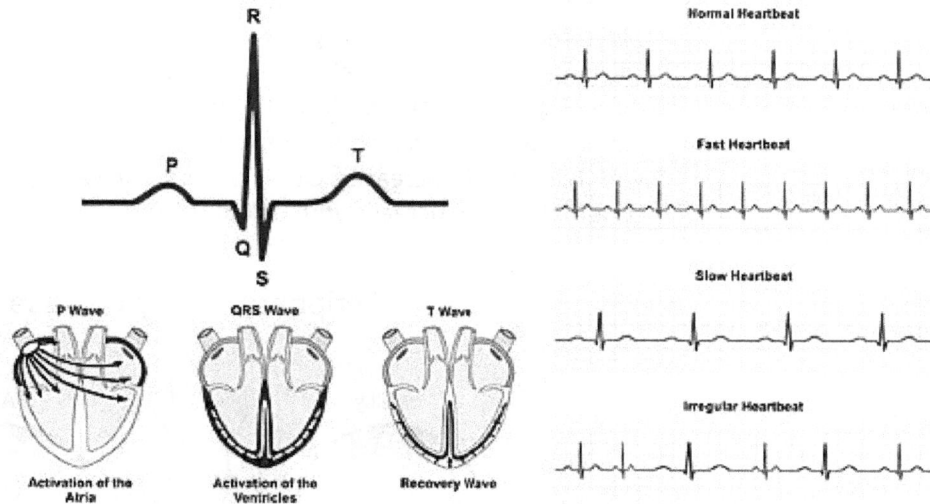

Although palpitations are very common and usually harmless, they can be frightening when they happen and may cause anxiety.

- Most go away on their own.
- To prevent palpitations, you can try to avoid things that trigger them, such as stress, alcohol, or caffeine.
- You also may prevent palpitations by treating any other medical condition that may be causing them.

**Palpitations may be a sign of more serious heart problems.**

- You should seek medical attention immediately if you have palpitations and feel dizzy or confused, have trouble breathing, thinking you may faint, or have pain or tightness in your chest.

*Peripheral Arterial Disease (PAD)*

*AKA*
*\*Atherosclerotic peripheral arterial disease*

*\*Claudication*

*\*Hardening of the arteries*

*\*Leg cramps from poor circulation*

*\*Peripheral arterial disease*

*\*Peripheral vascular disease*

*\*Poor circulation*

*\*Vascular disease*

*CDC,*
*NIH PAD and Cinahl Information Systems*

**Peripheral Arterial Disease (PAD)**
Occurs when the arteries that supply blood to the arms and legs (the periphery) become narrow or stiff. PAD usually results from atherosclerosis, the buildup of plaque and narrowing of the arteries. With this condition, blood flow and oxygen to the arm and leg muscles are low or even fully blocked.

**Signs and symptoms** include leg pain, numbness, and swelling in the ankles and feet.
- Blocked blood flow to your legs can cause pain and numbness. It also can raise your risk of getting an infection in the affected limbs. Your body may have a hard time fighting the infection.
- If severe enough, blocked blood flow can cause gangrene (tissue death). In very serious cases, this can lead to leg amputation.
- If you have leg pain when you walk or climb stairs, talk with your doctor. Sometimes older people think that leg pain is just a symptom of aging, however, the cause of the pain could be PAD. Tell your doctor if you are feeling pain in your legs and discuss whether you should be tested for PAD.
- Smoking is the main risk factor for PAD. If you smoke or have a history of smoking, your risk of PAD increases. Other factors, such as age and having certain diseases or conditions, also increase your risk of PAD.

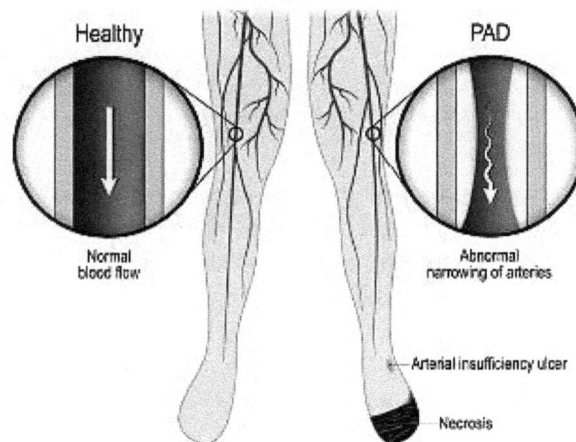

Peripheral artery disease

**The most common cause of peripheral artery disease (PAD.) is *atherosclerosis*.**
The disease may start if certain factors damage the inner layers of the arteries. These factors include:
- Smoking
- High amounts of certain fats and cholesterol in the blood
- High blood pressure
- High amounts of sugar in the blood due to insulin resistance or diabetes

**When damage occurs, your body starts a healing process.**
- The healing may cause plaque to build up where the arteries are damaged.
- Eventually, a section of plaque can rupture (break open), causing a blood clot to form at the site.
- The buildup of plaque or blood clots can severely narrow or block the arteries and limit the flow of oxygen-rich blood to your body.

| | |
|---|---|
| *Peripheral Arterial Disease (PAD)*<br><br>*Continued*<br><br>*Signs* and *Symptoms*<br><br>*Exercise* and *Precautions* | **Presentation/signs and symptoms**<br>Patients might present with a history of chronic and reproducible activity-related intermittent claudication (IC).<br>• Described as burning, heaviness/deep fatigue, and/or cramping in the legs<br>• Onset often begins in the calf muscles<br>• Bilateral or unilateral<br>• Pain might extend to proximal leg muscles (thigh and buttock) in severe cases<br>• Pain is relieved by slowing or stopping the activity<br>• Only present in 10% of patients with PAD; in fact, the American Heart Association estimates that 75% of the 8-12 million Americans with PAD are asymptomatic<br>• The intensity of IC pain typically increases with the intensity/speed and distance of leg exercise such as walking or cycling<br>• Weak lower extremity pulses and ABI ≤ 90<br>• Bruit (i.e., vascular sound heard through auscultation when blood flow is abnormal) might be present over carotid arteries, abdominal aorta, and iliac and femoral arteries<br>• Patient might also present with resting leg pain, non-healing wounds, and impotence/erectile dysfunction<br><br>**Living With Peripheral Artery Disease Symptoms** *(Cinahl Information Systems)*<br>• If you have PAD., you may feel pain in your calf or thigh muscles after walking. Try to take a break and allow the pain to ease before walking again. Over time, this may increase the distance that you can walk without pain.<br>• Talk with your doctor about taking part in a supervised exercise program. This type of program has been shown to reduce PAD symptoms.<br>• Check your feet and toes regularly for sores or possible infections. Wear comfortable shoes that fit well. Maintain good foot hygiene and have professional medical treatment for corns, bunions, or calluses.<br><br>**Exercise and/or Precautions**<br>Overall Contraindications/Precautions *(Cinahl Information Systems)*<br>• Obtain physician clearance for patient to participate in individualized exercise training program; adhere to any parameters set by the physician for vitals and exercise intensity.<br>• Deep vein thrombosis (DVT) with or without critical limb ischemia contraindicates exercise.<br>• Acute limb ischemia is a medical emergency, and any patient suspected of having this (*see symptoms listed above, under* Description) should be immediately referred to emergency services.<br>• Ischemic leg pain at rest is a relative contraindication to exercise.<br>   o However, critical limb ischemia should be immediately ruled out (especially in patients with diabetes, neuropathy, chronic renal failure, or limb infection) as risk of amputation is high.<br>• Multiple precautions might be warranted depending on any existing comorbidities, scope of disabilities, and weight-bearing restrictions from physician. |

| | |
|---|---|
| **Pacemaker** <br><br> *NIH* <br> *and* <br> *LiveStrong - Pacemakers* | A pacemaker is a small device that is placed in the chest or abdomen to help control abnormal heart rhythms. This device uses electrical pulses to prompt the heart to beat at a normal rate. <br> • Used to treat *arrhythmias*. During an arrhythmia, the heart can beat too fast, too slow, or with an irregular rhythm. <br> • A heartbeat that is too fast is called ***tachycardia***. <br> • A heartbeat that is too slow is called ***bradycardia***. <br> • During an ***arrhythmia***, the heart may not be able to pump enough blood to the body. This can cause symptoms such as fatigue (tiredness), shortness of breath, or fainting. Severe arrhythmias can damage the body's vital organs and may even cause loss of consciousness or death. <br> • A pacemaker can relieve some symptoms of arrhythmia, such as fatigue and fainting. <br> • A pacemaker also can help a person who has abnormal heart rhythms resume a more active lifestyle. <br><br> 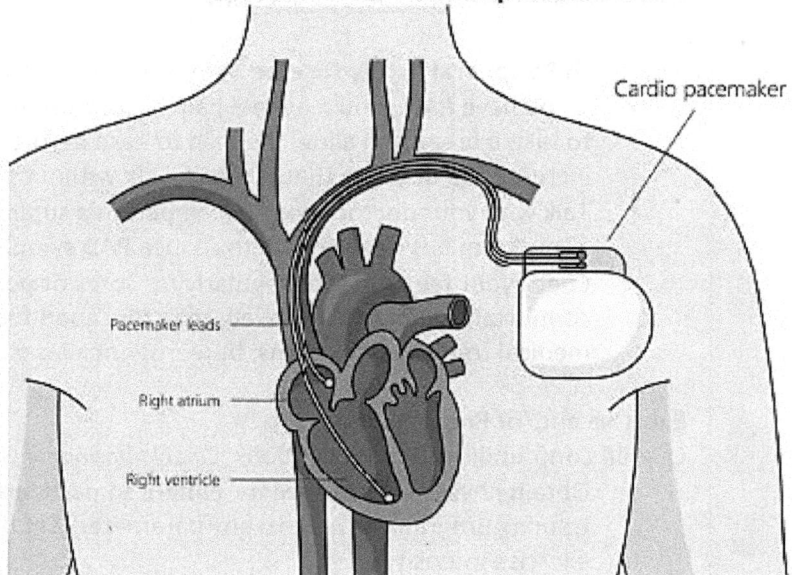 <br> Artificial cardiac pacemaker <br><br> Once you have a pacemaker, you must avoid close or prolonged contact with electrical devices or devices that have strong magnetic fields. <br><br> Devices that can interfere with a pacemaker include: <br> • Cell phones and MP3 players (for example, iPods) <br> • Household appliances, such as microwave ovens <br> • High-tension wires <br> • Metal detectors <br> • Industrial welders <br> • Electrical generators |

| | |
|---|---|
| **Pacemaker**<br><br>*Continued*<br><br>***Exercise* and Precautions**<br><br>*Livestrong – Exercise and Precautions* | These devices can disrupt the electrical signaling of your pacemaker and stop it from working properly. You may not be able to tell whether your pacemaker has been affected.<br>• How likely a device is to disrupt your pacemaker depends on how long you are exposed to it and how close it is to your pacemaker.<br>• To be safe, some experts recommend not putting your cell phone or MP3 player in a shirt pocket over your pacemaker (if the devices are turned on).<br>• You may want to hold your cell phone up to the ear that is opposite the site where your pacemaker is implanted. If you strap your MP3 player to your arm while listening to it, put it on the arm that is farther from your pacemaker.<br>• You can still use household appliances, but avoid close and prolonged exposure, as it may interfere with your pacemaker.<br>• You can walk through security system metal detectors at your normal pace. Security staff can check you with a metal detector wand as long as it isn't held for too long over your pacemaker site. You should avoid sitting or standing close to a security system metal detector. Notify security staff if you have a pacemaker.<br>• Also, stay at least 2 feet away from industrial welders and electrical generators.<br><br>**Some medical procedures can disrupt your pacemaker.**<br>These procedures include:<br>• Magnetic resonance imaging, or MRI<br>• Shock-wave lithotripsy to get rid of kidney stones.<br>• Electrocauterization to stop bleeding during surgery.<br><br>Let all your doctors, dentists, and medical technicians know that you have a pacemaker.<br>• Your doctor can give you a card that states what kind of pacemaker you have.<br>• Carry this card in your wallet.<br>• You may want to wear a medical ID bracelet or necklace that states that you have a pacemaker.<br><br>**Exercise and/or Precautions**<br>• In most cases, having a pacemaker will not limit you from doing sports and exercise, including strenuous activities.<br>• Although there are not many limitations on exercise after a pacemaker, there are some, particularly in the first months after implantation.<br>    o According to Arrythmia.org, you should avoid exercises like golf, swimming, tennis, or other exercises involving extensive range of motion in the shoulders during the first six weeks after surgery.<br>    o You should also avoid heavy lifting during this time.<br>• According to Cardiac Athletes.org, contact sports are *not* suitable for a person with a pacemaker, as these sports may damage your pacemaker.<br>    o You should also take care, even after six weeks, when doing exercises requiring shoulder motion, as these may cause you to crush the pacemaker wire between your first rib and clavicle. *(LiveStrong)* |

| | |
|---|---|
| **Implantable Cardioverter Defibrillator (ICD)** *AKA* ***Cardiac implantable devices* or *Defibrillators*** *HealthLine* *See* ***Cardiomyopathy*** *for* ***Exercise and/or Precautions*** | An implantable cardioverter defibrillator (ICD) is a small device that your doctor can put into your chest to help regulate an irregular heart rhythm, or an arrhythmia.<br>• Although it is smaller than a deck of cards, the ICD contains a battery and a small computer that monitors your heart rate. The computer delivers small electrical shocks to your heart at certain moments. This helps control your heart rate.<br>• Doctors most commonly implant ICDs in people who have life-threatening arrhythmias and who are at risk for sudden cardiac arrest, a condition in which the heart stops beating.<br>• Arrhythmias can be congenital (something you were born with) or a symptom of heart disease. |

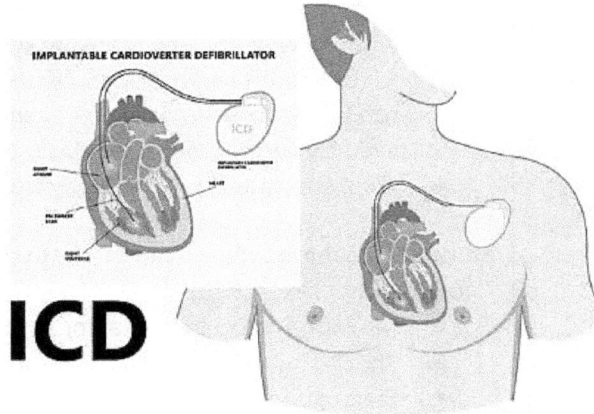

**You might benefit from an ICD if you have:**
- A very fast and dangerous heart rhythm called ventricular tachycardia.
- Erratic pumping, which is referred to as quivering or ventricular fibrillation.
- A heart weakened by a history of heart disease or a previous heart attack.
- An enlarged or thickened heart muscle, which is called dilated, or hypertrophic, cardiomyopathy.
- Congenital heart defects, such as long QT syndrome, which causes heart quivering.
- Heart failure

**An ICD can also deliver up to four types of electrical signals to your heart:**
- *Cardioversion*. Cardioversion gives a strong electrical signal that can feel like a thump to your chest. It resets heart rhythms to normal when it detects a very fast heart rate.
- *Defibrillation*. Defibrillation sends a very strong electrical signal that restarts your heart. The sensation is painful and can knock you off your feet but lasts only a second.
- *Anti-tachycardia pacing* provides a low-energy pulse meant to reset a rapid heartbeat. Typically, you feel nothing when the pulse occurs. However, you may sense a small flutter in your chest.
- *Bradycardia pacing* restores to normal speed a heartbeat that is too slow. In this situation, the ICD works like a pacemaker. People with ICDs usually have hearts that beat too fast. However, defibrillation can sometimes cause the heart to slow down to a dangerous level. Bradycardia pacing returns the rhythm to normal.

**Certain objects can interfere with your device's performance, so you will need to avoid them.**
- These include security systems, certain medical equipment, like MRI machines, power generators. You should also try to keep cell phones and other mobile devices at least six inches away from your ICD. (*also see Pacemakers*)

## Hypertension and Hypotension

### Hypertension

*AKA*
**High Blood Pressure**

*CDC
and
NIH- Blood
pressure*

High blood pressure usually has no warning signs or symptoms, so many people don't realize they have it. There is only one way to know whether you have high blood pressure: Have a doctor or other health professional measure it. Measuring your blood pressure is quick and painless.

***What Blood Pressure Numbers Mean?***
Blood pressure is measured using two numbers.
- The first number, called *systolic blood pressure*, represents the pressure in your blood vessels when your heart beats.
- The second number, called *diastolic blood pressure*, represents the pressure in your blood vessels when your heart rests between beats.
- Blood pressure is measured in millimeters of mercury (mmHg).

The chart below shows normal, at-risk, and high blood pressure levels. A blood pressure less than 120/80 mmHg is normal. A blood pressure of 140/90 mmHg or more is too high. People with levels from 120/80 mmHg to 139/89 mmHg have a condition called pre-hypertension, which means they are at high risk for high blood pressure.

**Blood Pressure Levels**
- **Normal**
  systolic: less than 120 mmHg
  diastolic: less than 80mmHg
- **At risk**
  (pre-hypertension)
  systolic: 120–139 mmHg
  diastolic: 80–89 mmHg
- **High**
  systolic: 140 mmHg or higher
  diastolic: 90 mmHg or higher

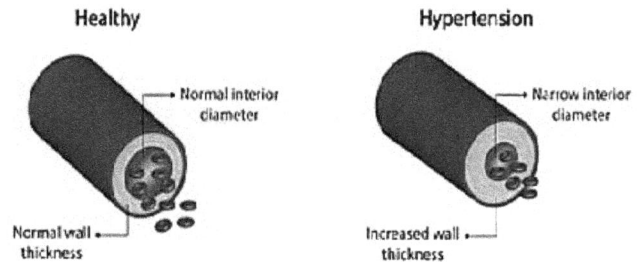

It is important to have regular blood pressure readings taken and to know your numbers, because high blood pressure usually does not cause symptoms until serious complications occur.

***Undiagnosed or uncontrolled high blood pressure can cause the following complications:***
- Aneurysms
- Chronic kidney disease
- Eye damage
- Heart attack
- Heart failure
- Peripheral artery disease
- Stroke
- Vascular dementia

***Controlling High Blood Pressure***
Keeping your blood pressure levels in a healthy range usually involves:
- Taking medications
- Heart-healthy eating
- Reducing sodium in the diet
- Getting daily physical activity
- Quitting smoking

| **Hypotension**<br><br>*NIH Hypotension* | **Hypotension is abnormally low blood pressure.**<br>• Blood pressure is the force of blood pushing against the walls of the arteries as the heart pumps out blood.<br>• Blood pressure is measured as systolic and diastolic pressures. "Systolic" refers to blood pressure when the heart beats while pumping blood. "Diastolic" refers to blood pressure when the heart is at rest between beats. *(See Hypertension above)*<br><br>**There are several types of hypotension.**<br>People who always have low blood pressure have chronic asymptomatic hypotension.<br>• They usually have no signs or symptoms and need no treatment.<br>• Their low blood pressure is normal for them.<br>• The **three main types** of this kind of hypotension are ***orthostatic hypotension, neurally mediated hypotension,*** and ***severe hypotension linked to shock.***<br><br>**Orthostatic Hypotension.** The signs and symptoms of orthostatic hypotension and neurally mediated hypotension (NMH) are similar. They include:<br>   ○ Dizziness or light-headedness<br>   ○ Blurry vision<br>   ○ Confusion<br>   ○ Weakness<br>   ○ Fatigue (feeling tired)<br>   ○ Nausea (feeling sick to your stomach)<br><br>This type of hypotension occurs when standing up from a sitting or lying down position. You may feel dizzy or light-headed, or you may even faint.<br>• Orthostatic hypotension occurs if your body isn't able to adjust blood pressure and blood flow fast enough for the change in position.<br>   ○ The drop in blood pressure usually lasts only for a few seconds or minutes after you stand up. You may need to sit or lie down for a short time while your blood pressure returns to normal.<br>• Orthostatic hypotension can occur in all age groups; however, it is more common in older adults, especially those who are frail or in poor health.<br>   ○ This type of hypotension can be a symptom of another medical condition. Thus, treatment often focuses on treating underlying conditions.<br>• Some people also have high blood pressure when lying down.<br>• A form of orthostatic hypotension called ***postprandial hypotension*** is a sudden drop in blood pressure after a meal. This type of hypotension mostly affects older adults.<br>   ○ People who have high blood pressure or a central nervous system disorder, such as Parkinson's disease, also are at increased risk for postprandial hypotension.<br><br>**Neurally Mediated Hypotension**<br>• See *Orthostatic* above for signs and symptoms.<br>• With neurally mediated hypotension (NMH), blood pressure drops after you've been standing for a long time. You may feel dizzy, faint, or sick to the stomach as a result.<br>• NMH also can occur as the result of an unpleasant, upsetting, or scary situation.<br>• NMH affects children and young adults more often than people in other age groups. Children often outgrow NMH.<br><br>**Severe Hypotension Linked to Shock**<br>• Shock is a life-threatening condition in which blood pressure drops so low that the brain, kidneys, and other vital organs can't get enough blood to work well.<br>• Blood pressure drops much lower in shock than in other types of hypotension.<br>• Many factors can cause shock. Examples include major blood loss, certain severe infections, severe burns and allergic reactions, and poisoning.<br>   ○ Shock can be fatal if it'snot treated right away. |

**Hypotension**

*Continued*

*Shock – Signs and Symptoms*

*Living with Hypotension*

**Signs and Symptoms**

- In shock, not enough blood and oxygen flow to the body's major organs, including the brain. The early signs and symptoms of reduced blood flow to the brain include light-headedness, sleepiness, and confusion.
- In the earliest stages of shock, it may be hard to detect any signs or symptoms. In older people, the first symptom may only be confusion.
- Over time, as shock worsens, a person won't be able to sit up without passing out. If the shock continues, the person will lose consciousness. Shock often is fatal if not treated right away.
- Other signs and symptoms of shock vary, depending on what's causing the shock. When low blood volume (from major blood loss, for example) or poor pumping action in the heart (from heart failure, for example) causes shock:
  - The skin becomes cold and sweaty. It often looks blue or pale. If pressed, the color returns to normal more slowly than usual. A bluish network of lines appears under the skin.
  - The pulse becomes weak and rapid.
  - The person begins to breathe very quickly.
- When extreme relaxation of blood vessels causes shock (such as in **vasodilatory shock**), a person feels warm and flushed at first. Later, the skin becomes cold and sweaty, and the person feels very sleepy.
- Shock is an emergency and must be treated right away. If a person has signs or symptoms of shock, call 9–1–1.

**Living with Hypotension**

- Doctors can successfully treat hypotension. Many people who had the condition and were successfully treated live normal, healthy lives.
- If you have hypotension, you can take steps to prevent or limit symptoms, such as dizzy spells and fainting.
- If you have *orthostatic hypotension,* get up slowly after sitting or lying down, or move your legs before changing your position.
- Eat small, low-carbohydrate meals if you have *postprandial hypotension* (a form of orthostatic hypotension).
- If you have *neurally mediated hypotension*, try not to stand for long periods. If you do have to stand for a long time, move around and wear compression stockings. These stockings apply pressure to your lower legs. The pressure helps move blood throughout your body.
- Drink plenty of fluids, such as water or sport drinks that contain nutrients like sodium and potassium. Also, try to avoid unpleasant, upsetting, or scary situations. Learn to recognize symptoms and take action to raise your blood pressure.
- Ask your doctor about learning how to measure your own blood pressure. This will help you find out what a normal blood pressure reading is for you. Keeping a record of blood pressure readings done by health providers also can help you learn more about your blood pressure.
- ***Severe hypotension linked to shock is an emergency***. Shock can lead to death if it's not treated right away. If you see someone having signs or symptoms of shock, call 911.
  - Signs and symptoms of shock include light-headedness, sleepiness, and confusion. Over time, as shock worsens, a person won't be able to sit up without passing out. If the shock continues, the person can lose consciousness.
  - Other signs and symptoms of shock include cold and sweaty skin, a weak and rapid pulse, and rapid breathing.

## Cholesterol and Triglycerides

**Cholesterol**

*CDC - Cholesterol*

Cholesterol travels through the blood on proteins called "lipoproteins." Two types of lipoproteins carry cholesterol throughout the body:

- **LDL** (low-density lipoprotein), sometimes called *"bad"* cholesterol, makes up most of your body's cholesterol. High levels of LDL cholesterol raise your risk for heart disease and stroke.
- **HDL** (high-density lipoprotein), or *"good"* cholesterol, absorbs cholesterol and carries it back to the liver. The liver then flushes it from the body. High levels of HDL cholesterol can lower your risk for heart disease and stroke.

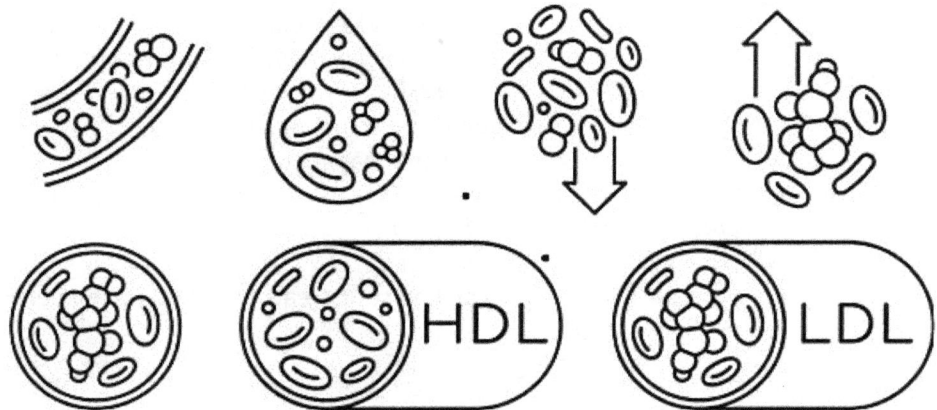

When your body has too much LDL cholesterol, the LDL cholesterol can build up on the walls of your blood vessels. This buildup is called "plaque."

- As your blood vessels build up plaque over time, the insides of the vessels narrow. This narrowing blocks blood flow to and from your heart and other organs.
- When blood flow to the heart is blocked, it can cause angina (chest pain) or a heart attack.
- Overweight and obesity raise levels of LDL ("bad") cholesterol. Excess body fat affects how your body uses cholesterol and slows down your body's ability to remove LDL cholesterol from your blood. The combination raises your risk of heart disease and stroke.

**There are two sources of cholesterol**: cholesterol made by the body and dietary cholesterol.

- *Body*: Cholesterol is made in your liver. Your body uses cholesterol to make hormones and digest fatty foods. Your body makes all the cholesterol it needs.
- *Dietary* cholesterol is in animal foods, such as egg yolks, fatty meats, and regular cheese. In general, foods that are high in dietary cholesterol are also high in saturated fat.

**Lowering Your Risk**

- If you have *high LDL* cholesterol levels, your health care team may recommend cholesterol-lowering medicine and lifestyle changes to lower your risk for heart disease and stroke.
- If you have *low HDL* cholesterol levels, talk to your doctor about lifestyle changes that may help raise your levels.

Your body makes all of the cholesterol it needs, so you do not need to obtain cholesterol through foods.

- Eating lots of foods high in saturated fat and trans-fat may contribute to high cholesterol and related conditions, such as heart disease.

| Cholesterol<br><br>*Continued*<br><br><br>*What you can do*<br><br>*Medications* | **What you can do:** |
|---|---|

**What you can do:**
- Limit foods high in saturated fat. Saturated fats come from animal products (such as cheese, fatty meats, and dairy desserts) and tropical oils (such as palm oil).
  - Foods that are higher in saturated fat may be high in cholesterol.
- Choose foods that are low in saturated fat, trans fat, sodium (salt), and added sugars.
  - These foods include lean meats; seafood; fat-free or low-fat milk, cheese, and yogurt;whole grains; and fruits and vegetables.
- Eat foods naturally high in fiber, such as oatmeal and beans (black, pinto, kidney, Lima, and others) and unsaturated fats, which can be found in avocado, vegetable oils like olive oil and nuts).
  - These foods may help prevent and manage high levels of low-density lipoprotein (LDL, or "bad") cholesterol and triglycerides while increasing high-density lipoprotein (HDL, or "good") cholesterol levels.
- Physical activity can help you maintain a healthy weight and lower your cholesterol and blood pressure levels.
- Smoking damages your blood vessels, speeds up the hardening of the arteries, and greatly increases your risk for heart disease. If you do smoke, quitting will lower your risk for heart disease.
- Too much alcohol can raise cholesterol levels and the levels of triglycerides, a type of fat in the blood. Avoid drinking too much alcohol. Men should have no more than two drinks per day, and women should have no more than one.

**Types of Cholesterol-lowering Medicine**
Several types of medicines help lower LDL cholesterol. The chart below describes each type and how it works.

**Types of Medicine**
- *Statin drugs* lower LDL cholesterol by slowing down the liver's production of cholesterol. They also increase the liver's ability to remove LDL cholesterol that is already in the blood.
- *Bile acid sequestrants* help remove cholesterol from the blood stream by removing bile acids. The body needs bile acids and makes them by breaking down LDL cholesterol.
- **Niacin or nicotinic acid**. Niacin is a B vitamin that can improve all lipoprotein levels. Nicotinic acid raises high-density lipoprotein (HDL) cholesterol levels while lowering total cholesterol, LDL cholesterol, and triglyceride levels.
- **Fibrates** mainly lower triglycerides.
- **Injectable medicine**. A newer type of medicine called PCSK9 inhibitors lowers cholesterol. These medicines are primarily used in people who have familial hypercholesterolemia, a genetic condition that causes very high levels of LDL cholesterol.

All drugs may have side effects, so talk with your health care team, including your pharmacist, on a regular basis. Once your cholesterol levels have improved, your health care team will monitor them to ensure they stay in a healthy range.

*Who Needs Cholesterol-lowering Medicine?*
Your treatment plan for high cholesterol will depend on your current cholesterol levels and your risk of heart disease and stroke.
- Your risk for heart disease and stroke depends on other risk factors, including high blood pressure and high blood pressure treatment, smoking status, age, high-density lipoprotein cholesterol level, total cholesterol level, diabetes, family history, and whether you have already had a heart attack or stroke.

**Your health care provider may prescribe medicine if:**
- You have already had a heart attack or stroke, or you have peripheral arterial disease.
- Your LDL cholesterol level is 190 mg/dL or higher.
- You are 40–75 years old with diabetes and an LDL cholesterol level of 70 mg/dL or higher.
- You are 40–75 years old with a high risk of developing heart disease or stroke and an LDL cholesterol level of 70 mg/dL or higher.

## Triglycerides
*(High Blood)*

*AKA*
***Hypertriglyceridemia***

***Dyslipidemia***

***Lipid Disorder***

*NIH - Triglycerides*

**High blood triglycerides are a type of lipid disorder, or dyslipidemia.**
- This condition may occur on its own, with other lipid disorders such as high blood cholesterol or low HDL cholesterol, or as part of metabolic syndrome.

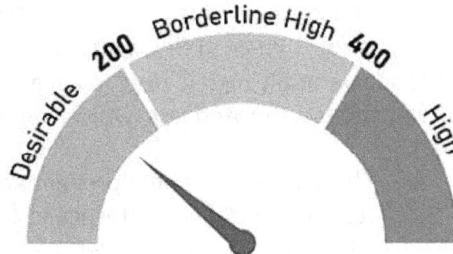

**Triglycerides (mg/dL)**

**Risk Factors**
Certain medical conditions, genetics, lifestyle habits, and some medicines are all risk factors for high blood triglycerides.
- Medical conditions that may increase blood triglyceride levels include thyroid disease, diabetes, liver and kidney diseases, and overweight and obesity.
- Sometimes the gene you inherited can cause high blood triglyceride levels.
- Being physically inactive, eating foods that are high in fat and sugar, or drinking too much alcohol may increase blood triglycerides.
- Some medicines used to treat breast cancer, high blood pressure, HIV, and other conditions may also increase triglyceride levels in the blood.

**High blood triglycerides usually do not cause any symptoms.**
- Untreated or uncontrolled high blood triglyceride levels may increase your risk of serious complications such as coronary heart disease and stroke.
- Very high blood triglycerides can increase the risk of acute pancreatitis, which is inflammation of the pancreas that causes severe pain in the abdomen.

Based on your risk factors and your personal and family health histories, your doctor may recommend testing you for high blood triglycerides with a routine blood test called a lipid panel.
- **A lipid panel** measures the total cholesterol, HDL cholesterol, LDL cholesterol, and triglyceride levels in your blood.
- Your doctor may diagnose you with high blood triglycerides if your fasting blood triglyceride levels are consistently 150 milligrams per deciliter (mg/dL) or higher.
- Normal fasting blood triglyceride levels are less than 75 mg/dLfor children under the age of 10 and less than 90 mg/dL for children aged 10 and older and adults.

If you are diagnosed with high blood triglycerides, your doctor may first recommend that you adopt heart-healthy lifestyle changes, such as healthy eating, which includes limiting alcohol, added sugars, and foods high in saturated or trans fats; getting regular physical activity; quitting smoking; and aiming for a healthy weight.
- Your doctor may also prescribe medicines such as fibrates, omega-3 fatty acids, nicotinic acid, or statins to control or lower your triglyceride levels.

# Stroke *aka* Cerebrovascular accident (CVA) & TIA's
### *CDC or NIH Stroke unless otherwise specified*

## *Quick Summary* of Section

### Understanding a Stroke
- A stroke, sometimes called a brain attack or CVA, occurs when something blocks blood supply to part of the brain or when a blood vessel in the brain bursts. In either case, parts of the brain become damaged or die.
- A stroke can cause lasting brain damage, long-term disability, or even death.

### Risk Factors
- Certain traits, conditions, and habits can raise your risk of having a stroke or transient ischemic attack (TIA). These traits, conditions, and habits are known as risk factors.
- The more risk factors you have, the more likely you are to have a stroke.

### Signs and Symptoms
- The signs and symptoms of a stroke often develop quickly. However, they can develop over hours or even days.
- The type of symptoms depends on the type of stroke and the area of the brain that is affected.

### Stroke Complications
- After you have had a stroke, you may develop other complications, such as: Blood Clots, Muscle Weakness, Pneumonia, Difficulty Swallowing, Loss of Bladder Control

### Hemorrhagic Stroke
- A hemorrhagic stroke happens when an artery in the brain leaks blood or ruptures (breaks open).
- The bleeding causes swelling of the brain and increased pressure in the skull.

### Transient Ischemic Attack (TIA) - Mini Stroke
- This is different from the major types of stroke because blood flow to the brain is blocked for only a short time—usually no more than 5 minutes.

### Mobility and Exercise after a Stroke
- A stroke can affect how well you sit, move, balance, stand and walk.
- Exercise will improve your fitness, your general health and reduce your risk of having another stroke

### Exercise and Stroke  (*National Stroke Association*)
- Movement, Paralysis, Spasticity and Exercise

## Stroke *aka* Cerebrovascular accident (CVA) & TIA's

**Stroke**

*AKA*
*\*Cerebrovascular accident (CVA)*

*\*Brain Attack*

*\* Hemorrhagic Stroke*

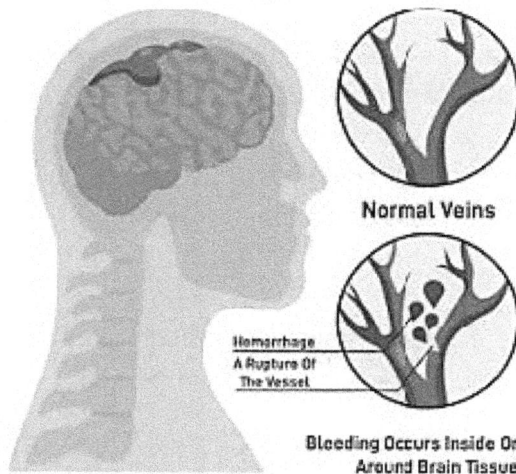

*\*Ischemic Stroke*

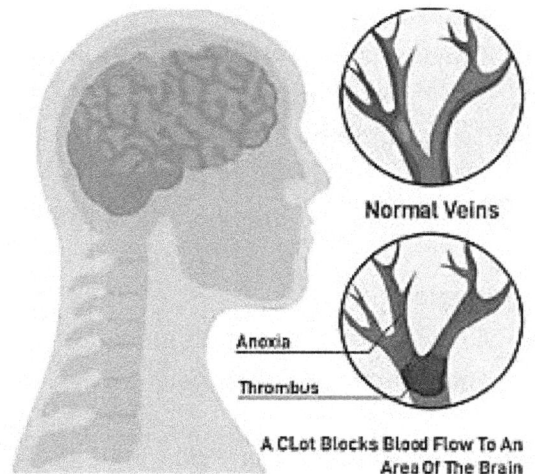

*CDC*
*and*
*NIH Stroke*

A stroke, sometimes called a brain attack or CVA, occurs when something blocks blood supply to part of the brain or when a blood vessel in the brain bursts.

- In either case, parts of the brain become damaged or die.
- A stroke can cause lasting brain damage, long-term disability, or even death.

**Understanding Stroke**
To understand stroke, it helps to understand the brain.

- The brain controls our movements, stores our memories, and is the source of our thoughts, emotions, and language.
- The brain also controls many functions of the body, like breathing and digestion.
- To work properly, your brain needs oxygen.
- Although your brain makes up only 2% of your body weight, it uses 20% of the oxygen you breathe. Your arteries deliver oxygen-rich blood to all parts of your brain.

# Types Of Stroke

### Hemorrhagic Stroke

Normal Veins

Hemorrhage
A Rupture Of
The Vessel

Bleeding Occurs Inside Or
Around Brain Tissue

### Ischemic Stroke

Normal Veins

Anoxia

Thrombus

A CLot Blocks Blood Flow To An
Area Of The Brain

**What Happens During a Stroke?**
If something happens to block the flow of blood, brain cells start to die within minutes because they cannot get oxygen. This causes a stroke.

There are two types of strokes:

- An *ischemic* stroke occurs when blood clots or other particles block the blood vessels to the brain. Fatty deposits called plaque can also cause blockages by building up in the blood vessels.
- A *hemorrhagic* stroke occurs when a blood vessel bursts in the brain. Blood builds up and damages surrounding brain tissue.

Both types of stroke damage brain cells.

- Symptoms of that damage start to show in the parts of the body controlled by those brain cells.

*See more below in next section on TIA/ Ischemic and hemorrhagic stroke.*

# Stroke

*Continued*

***Risk Factors***

***Risk Factors***

Certain traits, conditions, and habits can raise your risk of having a stroke or transient ischemic attack (TIA). These traits, conditions, and habits are known as risk factors.

- The more risk factors you have, the more likely you are to have a stroke.
- You can treat or control some risk factors, such as high blood pressure and smoking.
- Other risk factors, such as age and gender, you can't control.

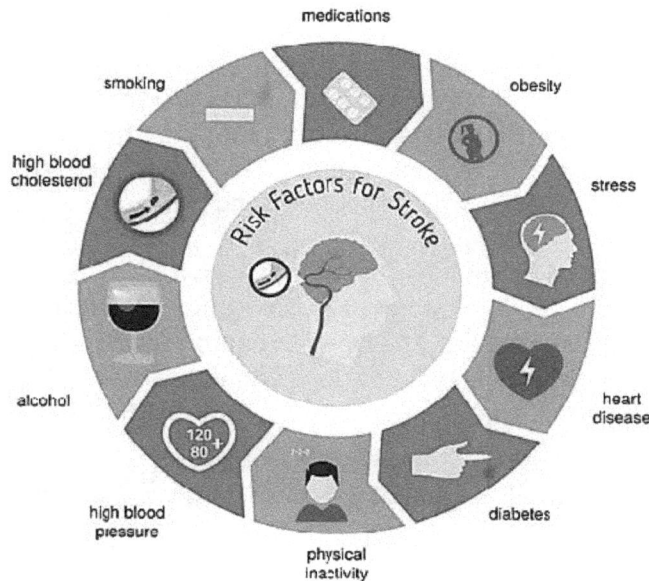

**The major risk factors for stroke include:**

- ***High blood pressure.*** High blood pressure is the main risk factor for stroke. Blood pressure is considered high if it stays at or above 140/90 millimeters of mercury (mmHg) over time. If you have diabetes or chronic kidney disease, high blood pressure is defined as 130/80 mmHg or higher.
- ***Diabetes.*** Diabetes is a disease in which the blood sugar level is high because the body doesn't make enough insulin or doesn't use its insulin properly. Insulin is a hormone that helps move blood sugar into cells where it's used for energy.
- ***Heart diseases.*** Coronary heart disease, cardiomyopathy, heart failure, and atrial fibrillation can cause blood clots that can lead to a stroke.
- ***Smoking.*** Smoking can damage blood vessels and raise blood pressure. Smoking also may reduce the amount of oxygen that reaches your body's tissues. Exposure to secondhand smoke also can damage the blood vessels.
- ***Age and gender***. Your risk of stroke increases as you get older. At younger ages, men are more likely than women to have strokes. However, women are more likely to die from strokes. Women who take birth control pills also are at slightly higher risk of stroke.
- ***Race and ethnicity***. Strokes occur more often in African American, Alaska Native, and American Indian adults than in white, Hispanic, or Asian American adults.
- ***Personal or family history of stroke or TIA***. If you've had a stroke, you're at higher risk for another one. Your risk of having a repeat stroke is the highest right after a stroke. A TIA also increases your risk of having a stroke, as does having a family history of stroke.
- ***Brain aneurysms or arteriovenous malformations (AVMs)***. Aneurysms are balloon-like bulges in an artery that can stretch and burst. AVMs are tangles of faulty arteries andveins that can rupture (break open) within the brain. AVMs may be present at birth but often aren't diagnosed until they rupture.

**Stroke**

*Continued*

***Risk Factors***

***Signs* and *Symptoms***

**Other risk factors for stroke, many of which of you can control, include:**
- Alcohol and illegal drug use, including cocaine, amphetamines, and other drugs
- Certain medical conditions, such as sickle cell disease, vasculitis (inflammation of the blood vessels), and bleeding disorders
- Lack of physical activity
- Overweight and Obesity
- Stress and depression
- Unhealthy cholesterol levels
- Unhealthy diet
- Use of nonsteroidal anti-inflammatory drugs (NSAIDs), but not aspirin, may increase the risk of heart attack or stroke, particularly in patients who have had a heart attack or cardiac bypass surgery. The risk may increase the longer NSAIDs are used. Common NSAIDs include ibuprofen and naproxen.

### Signs and Symptoms

The signs and symptoms of a stroke often develop quickly. However, they can develop over hours or even days. The type of symptoms depends on the type of stroke and the area of the brain that is affected. How long symptoms last and how severe they are vary among different people.

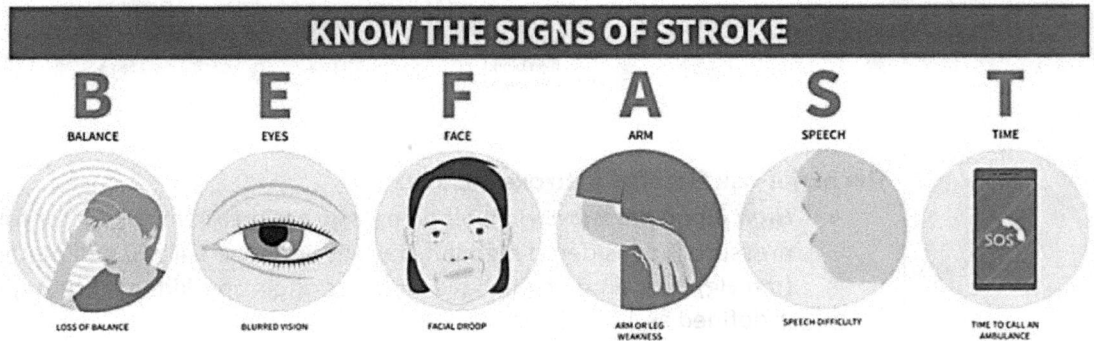

**KNOW THE SIGNS OF STROKE**

B — BALANCE — LOSS OF BALANCE
E — EYES — BLURRED VISION
F — FACE — FACIAL DROOP
A — ARM — ARM OR LEG WEAKNESS
S — SPEECH — SPEECH DIFFICULTY
T — TIME — TIME TO CALL AN AMBULANCE

**Signs and symptoms of a stroke may include:**
- Sudden weakness
- Paralysis (an inability to move) or numbness of the face, arms, or legs, especially on one side of the body
- Confusion
- Trouble speaking or understanding speech
- Trouble seeing in one or both eyes
- Problems breathing
- Dizziness, trouble walking, loss of balance or coordination, and unexplained falls
- Loss of consciousness
- Sudden and severe headache
- A transient ischemic attack (TIA) has the same signs and symptoms as a stroke. However, TIA symptoms usually last less than 1–2 hours (although they may last up to 24 hours). A TIA may occur only once in a person's lifetime or more often.

At first, it may not be possible to tell whether someone is having a TIA or stroke.
- All stroke-like symptoms require medical care.
- If you think you or someone else is having a TIA or stroke, call 9–1–1 right away. Do not drive to the hospital or let someone else drive you.
- Call an ambulance so that medical personnel can begin life-saving treatment on the way to the emergency room. During a stroke, every minute counts.

**Stroke**

*Continued*

**Complications**

### Stroke Complications

After you have had a stroke, you may develop other complications, such as:

- Blood clots and muscle weakness.
    - Being immobile (unable to move around) for a longtime can raise your risk of developing blood clots in the deep veins of the legs.
    - Being immobile also can lead to muscle weakness and decreased muscle flexibility.
- Problems swallowing and pneumonia.
    - If a stroke affects the muscles used for swallowing, you may have a hard time eating or drinking.
    - You also may be at risk of inhaling food or drink into your lungs.
    - If this happens, you may develop pneumonia.
- Loss of bladder control.
    - Some strokes affect the muscles used to urinate. You may need a urinary catheter (a tube placed into the bladder) until you can urinate on your own.
    - Use of these catheters can lead to urinary tract infections.
    - Loss of bowel controlor constipation also may occur after a stroke.

### Treating Stroke Risk Factors

After initial treatment for a stroke or TIA, your doctor will treat your risk factors. He or she mayrecommend heart-healthy lifestyle changes to help control your risk factors. Heart-healthy lifestyle changes may include:

- Heart-healthy eating
- Aiming for a healthy weight
- Managing stress
- Physical activity
- Quitting smoking
- If heart-healthy lifestyle changes are not enough, you may need medicine to control your risk factors.

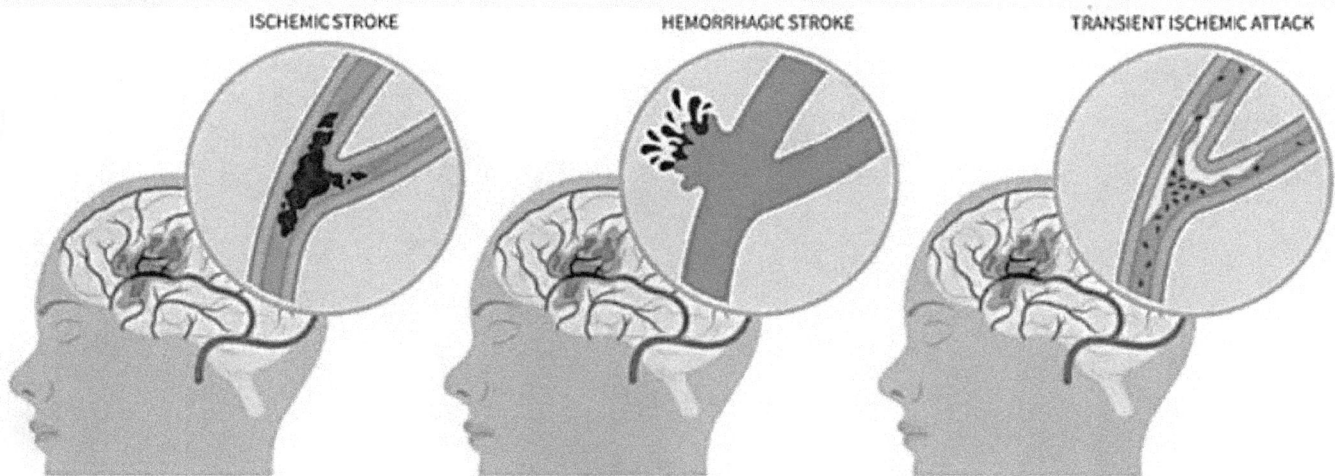

ISCHEMIC STROKE    HEMORRHAGIC STROKE    TRANSIENT ISCHEMIC ATTACK

# TYPES OF STROKE

| | |
|---|---|
| **HEMORRHAGIC STROKE** | A hemorrhagic stroke happens when an artery in the brain leaks blood or ruptures (breaks open).<br>• The bleeding causes swelling of the brain and increased pressure in the skull.<br>• The leaked blood puts too much pressure on brain cells, which damages them.<br>• High blood pressure and aneurysms—balloon-like bulges in an artery that can stretch and burst—are examples of conditions that can cause a hemorrhagic stroke.<br><br>There are two types of hemorrhagic strokes:<br>• **Intracerebral hemorrhage** is the most common type of hemorrhagic stroke.<br>   ○ It occurs when an artery in the brain bursts, flooding the surrounding tissue with blood.<br>• **Subarachnoid hemorrhage** is a less common type of hemorrhagic stroke.<br>   ○ It refers to bleeding in the area between the brain and the thin tissues that cover it.<br><br>Examples of conditions that can cause a hemorrhagic stroke include high blood pressure, aneurysms, and arteriovenous malformations (AVMs).<br>• **"Blood pressure"** is the force of blood pushing against the walls of the arteries as the heart pumps blood. If blood pressure rises and stays high over time, it can damage the body in many ways.<br>• **Aneurysms** are balloon-like bulges in an artery that can stretch and burst. AVMs are tangles of faulty arteries and veins that can rupture within the brain. High blood pressure can increase the risk of hemorrhagic stroke in people who have aneurysms or AVMs. |
| **TRANSIENT ISCHEMIC ATTACK (TIA)**<br><br>*AKA*<br>**Mini-Stroke** | A transient ischemic attack (TIA) is sometimes called a "mini-stroke." It is different from the major types of strokes because blood flow to the brain is blocked for only a short time—usually no more than 5 minutes.<br>• Most strokes (87%) are ischemic strokes.<br>• An ischemic stroke happens when blood flow through the artery that supplies oxygen-rich blood to the brain becomes blocked.<br>• Blood clots often cause the blockages that lead to ischemic strokes.<br><br>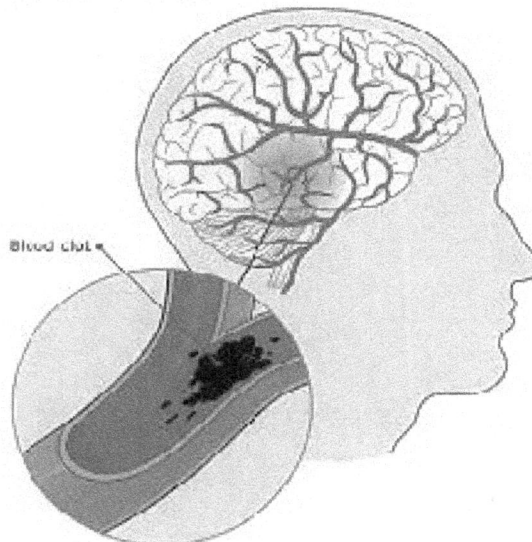<br>Transient ischemic attack |

| | |
|---|---|
| **TRANSIENT ISCHEMIC ATTACK (TIA)**<br><br>*Continued* | **Ischemic Stroke and Transient Ischemic Attack**<br><ul><li>An ischemic stroke or transient ischemic attack (TIA) occurs if an artery that supplies oxygen-rich blood to the brain becomes blocked. Many medical conditions can increase the risk of ischemic stroke or TIA.</li><li>For example, atherosclerosis is a disease in which a fatty substance called plaque builds up on the inner walls of the arteries. Plaque hardens and narrows the arteries, which limits the flow of blood to tissues and organs (such as the heart and brain).</li><li>Plaque in an artery can crack or rupture (break open). Blood platelets, which are disc-shaped cell fragments, stick to the site of the plaque injury and clump together to form blood clots. These clots can partly or fully block an artery.</li><li>Plaque can build up in any artery in the body, including arteries in the heart, brain, and neck. The two main arteries on each side of the neck are called the carotid arteries. These arteries supply oxygen-rich blood to the brain, face, scalp, and neck.</li><li>When plaque builds up in the carotid arteries, the condition is called carotid artery disease. Carotid artery disease causes many of the ischemic strokes and TIAs that occur in the United States.</li><li>An embolic stroke (a type of ischemic stroke) or TIA also can occur if a blood clot or piece of plaque breaks away from the wall of an artery. The clot or plaque can travel through the bloodstream and get stuck in one of the brain's arteries. This stops blood flow through the artery and damages brain cells.</li><li>Heart conditions and blood disorders also can cause blood clots that can lead to a stroke or TIA. For example, atrial fibrillation, or A-Fib, is a common cause of embolic stroke.</li><li>In A-Fib, the upper chambers of the heart contract in a very fast and irregular way. As a result, some blood pools in the heart. The pooling increases the risk of blood clots forming in the heart chambers.</li></ul><br>**It is important to know that:**<br><ul><li>A TIA is a warning sign of a future stroke.</li><li>A TIA is a medical emergency, just like a major stroke.</li><li>Strokes and TIAs require emergency care. Call 9-1-1 right away if you feel signs of a stroke or see symptoms in someone around you.</li><li>There is no way to know in the beginning whether symptoms are from a TIA or from a major type of stroke. Like ischemic strokes, blood clots often cause TIAs.</li><li>More than a third of people who have a TIA and don't get treatment have a major stroke within 1 year. As many as 10% to 15% of people will have a major stroke within 3 months of a TIA.</li><li>Recognizing and treating TIAs can lower the risk of a major stroke. If you have a TIA, your health care team can find the cause and take steps to prevent a major stroke.</li></ul> |

| | |
|---|---|
| **Mobility and Exercise after a Stroke**<br><br>*Stroke Foundation*<br>*- Mobility and Exercise after Stroke fact sheet*<br>and<br>*NIH* | ### What you need to know<br>- A stroke can affect how well you sit, move, balance, stand and walk.<br>- Your physiotherapist will work with you to set goals and develop a rehabilitation program to meet your needs.<br>- Exercise will improve your fitness, your general health and reduce your risk of having another stroke.<br><br>### How a stroke can affect mobility<br>**After a stroke, you may experience:**<br>- ***Weakness***. Your foot and leg may be paralyzed completely, or they may be weak. Paralysis on one side of the body is called hemiplegia. Weakness on one side of the body is called hemiparesis.<br>- ***Planning or coordinating problems.*** You may have difficulty planning leg movements. This is called *apraxia*. You may also have difficulty coordinating movements which makes them feel slow or clumsy. This is called *ataxia.*<br>- ***Changes in the muscles***. You may have high tone which makes your muscles stiff and tight. This is called *hypertonia* or *spasticity*. Alternatively, your muscles may be floppy or loose. This is called low tone or *hypotonia*.<br>- ***Balance.*** You may have difficulty keeping your balance, feel unsteady or dizzy.<br>- ***Contracture***. If your muscles are tight or weak, they can become shorter. This can result in the joint becoming fixed in one position.<br>- ***Changes in sensation.*** You might lose feeling, have pins and needles or have increased feeling *(hypersensitivity)*.<br>- ***Swelling***. If your leg or foot does not move as well as it used to, fluid may build up.<br>- ***Fatigue***. You may feel very tired after walking even a short distance. This is made worse because as you may have to concentrate hard on even simplest movements.<br>- ***Pain***. You may experience pain in your leg after a stroke, most often in the hip. This can make walking more difficult.<br><br>### Rehabilitation after Stroke *(NIH Stroke)*<br>After a stroke, you may need rehabilitation (rehab) to help you recover.<br>Rehab may include working with speech, physical, and occupational therapists.<br>- ***Language, Speech, and Memory***. You may have trouble communicating after a stroke. You may not be able to find the right words, put complete sentences together, or put words together in a way that makes sense. You also may have problems with your memory and thinking clearly. These problems can be very frustrating. *Speech and language therapists* can help you learn ways to communicate again and improve your memory.<br>- ***Muscle and Nerve Problems***. A stroke may affect only one side of the body or part of one side. It can cause paralysis (an inability to move) or muscle weakness, which can put you at risk for falling. *Physical and occupational therapists* can help you strengthen and stretch your muscles. They also can help you relearn how to do daily activities, such as dressing, eating, and bathing.<br>- ***Bladder and Bowel Problems***. A stroke can affect the muscles and nerves that control the bladder and bowels. You may feel like you have to urinate often, even if your bladder isn't full. You may not be able to get to the bathroom in time. Medicines and a *bladder or bowel specialist* can help with these problems.<br>- ***Swallowing and Eating Problems***. You may have trouble swallowing after a stroke. Signs of this problem are coughing or choking during eating or coughing up food after eating. A *speech therapist* can help you with these issues. They may suggest changes to your diet, such as eating puréed (finely chopped) foods or drinking thick liquid. |

| | |
|---|---|
| **Mobility and Exercise after a Stroke**<br><br>*Continued*<br><br>***Treatment and Recovery***<br><br>*Stroke Foundation* | *Treatment and Recovery (Stroke Foundation)*<br><br>Mobility difficulties affect everyone differently.<br>• Your physiotherapist will assess how well you move, sit, stand and walk.<br>• They will then work with you to set goals and develop a rehabilitation program to meet your needs.<br><br>**Your rehabilitation will focus on your specific difficulties.**<br><br>You may need to relearn how to:<br>• Roll over in bed.<br>• Move from sitting to standing.<br>• Move from a bed to a chair or a toilet (transferring).<br>• Walk.<br>• Exercises<br>  ○ Specifically prescribed exercises can improve your strength, coordination, balance, sensation, or fitness. Often this can be done during daily activities such as standing or walking. This is known as task-specific activity and is the most effective way to improve.<br>  ○ Repetition is key to improvement, so you may do movements many times. Movement and exercises can help to reduce muscle stiffness and pain.<br>  ○ Electrical stimulation may be used to strengthen weak muscles. Equipment such as treadmills may also be used as part of your rehabilitation program. Your therapist may also recommend video games to help you practice.<br>  ○ Weakness and contracture can cause 'foot drop'. This is when the foot or ankle drops down when you lift your leg to take a step.<br>    ▪ A plastic brace known as an ankle-foot orthosis (AFO) may be used for foot drop. These braces support the foot and ankle to help minimize tripping and reduce fall risks.<br>  ○ While you may make the most improvement in the first six months, regular activity will help you to continue your recovery. If you have been experiencing fatigue, depression or pain since your stroke, regular exercise may help.<br>    ▪ Exercise improves your fitness, your general health and reduces your risk of having another stroke.<br>  ○ You could join a fitness center or an exercise group at your local community health center. Talk to your doctor or physiotherapist before beginning or changing an exercise program.<br><br>**Falls**<br>• After a stroke, you may be at increased risk of falling. Wear comfortable, firm-fitting, flat shoes with a low broad heel and soles that grip. Do not wear poorly fitted slippers or walk in socks.<br>• Your therapists can assess how safe you are in different situations, such as going up and down the stairs and walking outdoors.<br>• Your physiotherapist may advise you to use a walking frame, stick or wheelchair, and will make sure you are using it safely.<br>• Your occupational therapist may assess your home for hazards and suggest equipment to prevent falls, such as a handrail or shower chair. |

## Exercise and Stroke

The following section is from the *National Stroke Association:*

**Life After Stroke:** *stroke.org/en/life-after-stroke*

**Life After Stroke and Exercise:** *stroke.org/en/life-after-stroke/recovery/exercise*

**Life after Stroke and Exercise - PDF:** *stroke.org/en/-/media/Stroke-Files/Stroke-Resource-Center/Recovery/Patient-Focused/Exercise-After-Stroke.pdf?sc_lang=en*

| | |
|---|---|
| **Movement** | The most common physical effect of stroke is muscle weakness and having less control of an affected arm or leg. Survivors often work with therapists to restore strength and control through exercise programs. They also learn skills to deal with the loss of certain body movements. |
| **Paralysis** | Paralysis is the inability of muscle or group of muscles to move on their own. After stroke, signals from the brain to the muscles often don't work right. This is due to stroke damage to the brain. Thisdamage can cause an arm or leg to become paralyzed and/or to develop spasticity. |
| **Spasticity** | Spasticity is a condition where muscles are stiff and resist being stretched. It can be found throughoutthe body but may be most common in the arms, fingers or legs. Depending on where it occurs, it can result in an arm being pressed against the chest, a stiff knee or a pointed foot that interferes with walking. It can also be accompanied by painful muscle spasms.<br><br>**Treatment Options for Spasticity**<br>• Treatment for spasticity is often a combination of therapy and medicine. Therapy can include range-of motion exercises, gentle stretching, and splinting or casting.<br>• Medicine can treat the general effects of spasticity and act on multiple muscle groups.<br>• Injections of botulinum toxin can prevent the release of chemicals that cause muscle contraction.<br>• One form of treatment involves the delivery of a drug directly into the spinal fluid using a surgically placed pump.<br>• Surgery is the last option to treat spasticity. It can be done on the brain or the muscles and joints. Surgery may block pain and restore some movement. |
| **Exercise** | Walking, bending and stretching are forms of exercise that can help strengthen your body and keep it flexible.<br>• Mild exercise, which should be undertaken every day, can take the form of a short walk or a simple activity like sweeping the floor.<br>• Stretching exercises, such as extending the arms or bending the torso, should be done regularly.<br>• Moving weakened or paralyzed body parts can be done while seated or lying down.<br>• Swimming is another beneficial exercise if the pool is accessible, and a helper is available.<br>• Use an exercise program that is written down, with illustrations and guidelines for a helper if necessary.<br><br>*Fatigue*<br>Fatigue while exercising is to be expected. Like everyone else, you will have good and bad days.<br>• You can modify these programs to accommodate for fatigue or other conditions.<br>• Avoid overexertion and pain, however, some discomfort may be necessary to make progress. |

## Starting an Exercise Program

More Information from the **American Stroke Association: HOPE Recovery Guide** Chapter 7

*stroke.org/-/media/Stroke-Files/life%20after%20stroke/ASA_HOPE_Stroke_Recovery_Guide_122020.pdf*

Depending on the level of the stroke, you most likely have already participated in a rehab program and will continue advancing with the team's guidance. For those with a TIA or higher level strokes, you may be able to start a program as outlined in the second half of this book after speaking with your physician.

**Please consult with your physician or rehab team before starting any exercise program or change in diet.**
This book is for reference and does not substitute for advice by your doctor, as every person is different and may have comorbidities along with their primary disease.

# Cardiac Nutrition

## *Quick Summary* this Section

### Heart-healthy eating (NIH)
- Foods to eat in a Heart Healthy Diet

### Nutrients to Limit
- Sodium,
- Saturated and Trans Fats
- Added Sugars
- Alcohol

### DASH Diet
- Foods to Eat
- Foods to Avoid
- Questionable or Decrease Consumption
- Possible other Names to Avoid

### References

BEST FOOD FOR HEALTHY HEART

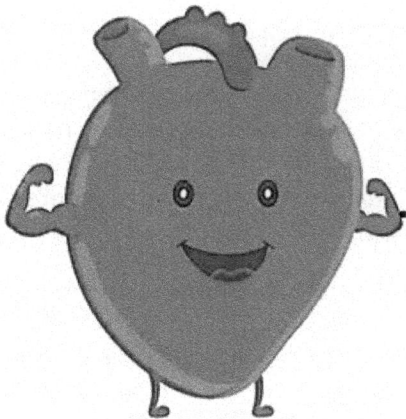

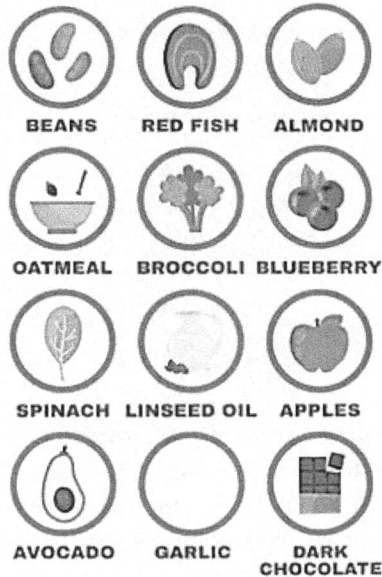

BEANS  RED FISH  ALMOND
OATMEAL  BROCCOLI  BLUEBERRY
SPINACH  LINSEED OIL  APPLES
AVOCADO  GARLIC  DARK CHOCOLATE

# Heart-healthy eating  (NIH)

| | |
|---|---|
| **Foods to Eat** | The following foods are the foundation of a heart-healthy diet.<br><br>• Vegetables such as greens (spinach, collard greens, kale), broccoli, cabbage, and carrots<br>• Fruits such as apples, bananas, oranges, pears, grapes, and prunes<br>• Whole grains such as plain oatmeal, brown rice, and whole-grain bread or tortillas<br>• Fat-free or low-fat dairy foods such as milk, cheese, or yogurt<br>• Protein-rich foods:<br>   o Fish high in omega-3 fatty acids, such as salmon, tuna, and trout, about 8 ounces a week<br>   o Lean meats such as 95 percent lean ground beef or pork tenderloin<br>   o Poultry such as skinless chicken or turkey<br>   o Eggs<br>   o Nuts, seeds, and soy products<br>   o Legumes such as kidney beans, lentils, chickpeas, black-eyed peas, and lima beans<br>• Oils and foods containing high levels of monounsaturated and polyunsaturated fats that can help lower blood cholesterol levels and the risk of cardiovascular disease. Some sources of these oils are:<br>   o Canola, corn, olive, safflower, sesame, sunflower, and soybean oils<br>   o Nuts such as walnuts, almonds, and pine nuts<br>   o Nut and seed butters<br>   o Salmon and trout<br>   o Seeds such as sesame, sunflower, pumpkin, or flax<br>   o Avocados<br>   o Tofu |
| **Nutrients to Limit** | **A heart-healthy diet limits sodium, saturated and trans fats, added sugars, and alcohol.**<br><br>### SODIUM<br><br>Adults and children over the age of 14 should eat less than 2,300 mg of sodium a day. Children younger than 14 may need to eat even less sodium each day based on their sex and age.<br>• If you have high blood pressure, you may need to restrict your sodium intake even more.<br>• Talk to yourdoctor or health care provider about what amount of sodium is right for you or your child.<br><br>**Try these shopping and cooking tips to help you choose and prepare foods that are lower in sodium.**<br>• Read food labels and choose products that have less sodium for the same serving size.<br>• Choose low-sodium, reduced sodium, or no-salt added products.<br>• Choose fresh, frozen, or no-salt-added foods instead of pre-seasoned, sauce-marinated, brined, or processed meats, poultry, and vegetables.<br>• Eat at home more often so you can cook food from scratch, which will allow you to control the amount of sodium in your meals.<br>• When cooking, limit your use of premade sauces, mixes, and "instant" products such as rice, noodles, and ready-made pasta.<br>• Flavor foods with herbs and spices instead of salt. |

| | |
|---|---|
| **Nutrients to Limit**<br><br>*Continued* | # SATURATED and TRANS FATS |

**When you follow a heart-healthy eating plan, you should:**
- Eat less than 10 percent of your daily calories from saturated fats found naturally in foods that come from animals and some plants.
- Limit intake of trans fats to as low as possible by limiting foods that contain high amounts of trans fats.

**The following are examples of foods that are high in saturated or trans fats.**
- Saturated fats are found in high amounts in fatty cuts of meat, poultry with skin, whole-milk dairy foods, butter, lard, and coconut and palm oils.
- Trans fats are found in high amounts in foods made with partially hydrogenated oils, such as some desserts, microwave popcorn, frozen pizza, stick margarines, and coffee creamers.

**To help you limit your intake of saturated fats and trans fats:**
- Read the nutrition labels and replace foods high in saturated fats with leaner, lower-fat animal products or vegetable oils, such as olive or canola oil instead of butter. Foods that are higher in saturated fats, such as fatty meats and high-fat dairy products, tend to be higher in dietary cholesterol that should also be limited.
- Read the nutrition labels and choose foods that do not contain trans fats. Some trans fats naturally occur in very small amounts in dairy products and meats. Foods containing these very low levels of natural trans fats do not need to be eliminated from your diet because they have other important nutrients.

| If you eat: | Try to eat no more than: |
|---|---|
| 1,200 calories a day | 8 grams of saturated fat a day |
| 1,500 calories a day | 10 grams of saturated fat a day |
| 1,800 calories a day | 12 grams of saturated fat a day |
| 2,000 calories a day | 13 grams of saturated fat a day |
| 2,500 calories a day | 17 grams of saturated fat a day |

Not all fats are bad. Monounsaturated and polyunsaturated fats actually help lower blood cholesterol levels.

**Some sources of monounsaturated and polyunsaturated fats are:**
- Avocados
- Corn, sunflower, and soybean oils
- Nuts and seeds, such as walnuts
- Olive, canola, peanut, safflower, and sesame oils
- Peanut butter
- Salmon and trout
- Tofu

**Nutrients
to Limit**

*Continued*

# Added SUGARS

- When you follow a heart-healthy eating plan, you should limit the amount of calories you consume each day from added sugars. Because added sugars do not provide essential nutrients and are extra calories, limiting them can help you choose nutrient-rich foods and stay within your daily calorie limit.
- Some foods, such as fruit, contain natural sugars. Added sugars do not occur naturally in foods but instead are used to sweeten foods and drinks.
  - Some examples of added sugarsinclude brown sugar, corn syrup, dextrose, fructose, glucose, high-fructose corn syrup, raw sugar, and sucrose.
- In the United States, sweetened drinks, snacks, and sweets are the major sources of added sugars. Sweetened drinks account for about half of all added sugars consumed. *The following are examples of foods and drinks with added sugars.*
  - Sweetened drinks include soft drinks or sodas, fruit drinks, sweetened coffee and tea, energy drinks, alcoholic drinks, and favored waters.
  - Snacks and sweets include grain-based desserts such as cakes, pies, cookies, brownies, doughnuts; dairy desserts such as ice cream, frozen desserts, and pudding; candies; sugars; jams; syrups; and sweet toppings.

**To help you reduce the amount of added sugars in your diet:**
- Choose unsweetened or whole fruits for snacks or dessert.
- Choose drinks without added sugar such as water, low-fat or fat-free milk, or 100 percent fruit or vegetable juice.
- Limit intake of sweetened drinks, snacks and desserts by eating them less often and in smaller amounts.

# ALCOHOL

If you drink alcohol, you should limit your intake. Men should have no more than two alcoholic drinks per day. Women should have no more than one alcoholic drink per day.
**One drink is:**
- 12 ounces of regular beer (5 percent alcohol)
- 5 ounces of wine (12 percent alcohol)
- 1½ ounces of 80-proof liquor (40 percent alcohol)

Talk to your doctor about how much alcohol you drink. Your doctor may recommend that you reduce the amount of alcohol you drink or that you stop drinking alcohol.
**Too much alcohol can:**
- Raise your blood pressure and levels of triglyceride fats in your blood.
- Add calories to your daily diet and possibly cause you to gain weight.
- Worsen heart failure in some patients.
- Contribute to heart failure in some people with cardiomyopathy.

**If you do not drink, you should not start drinking.**
- You should not drink if you are pregnant, underthe age of 21, taking certain medicines, or have certain medical conditions including heart failure.
- It is important for people with heart failure to take in the correct amounts and types of liquids because too much liquid can worsen heart failure.
- Remember that alcoholic drinks do contain calories and contribute to your daily calorie limits.The amount of calories will vary by the type of alcoholic drink.

| DASH Diet | Foods to Eat | Foods to avoid | Questionable or Decrease Consumption | Possible Other Names to Avoid |
|---|---|---|---|---|
| DASH stands for Dietary Approaches to Stop Hypertension. The DASH diet is a lifelong approach to healthy eating that's designed to help treat or prevent high blood pressure (hypertension). The DASH diet encourages you to reduce the sodium in your diet and eat a variety of foods rich in nutrients that help lower blood pressure, such as potassium, calcium, and magnesium.<br><br>*Mayo Clinic*<br><br>*Chewfo* | *Fruits.* Choose a variety of fresh fruits, such as apples, oranges and bananas. Add variety by looking beyond the ordinary to apricots, dates and berries. Select fruit canned in its own juice, not in heavy syrup, and frozen fruit without added sugar.<br><br>*Vegetables.* Buy fresh, frozen or canned vegetables, such as tomatoes, carrots, broccoli and spinach. Choose frozen vegetables without added salt or butter or sauces and opt for canned vegetables low in sodium.<br><br>*Low-fat dairy products.* Look for lower fat dairy options when buying milk, buttermilk, cheeses, yogurt and sour cream.<br><br>*Grains.* Aim for whole-grain and low-fat varieties of bread, bagels, pitas, cereal, rice, pasta, crackers and tortillas. Compare labels and choose the items lower in sodium.<br><br>*Nuts, seeds, and legumes.* Almonds, walnuts, kidney beans, lentils, chickpeas (garbanzos) and sunflower seeds are among the healthy options. But get the unsalted or low-salt varieties.<br><br>*Lean meats.* Poultry and fish. Opt for lean selections, such as fish, skinless chicken and turkey, pork tenderloin, extra-lean ground beef, and round or sirloin beef cuts. Avoid canned, smoked or processed meats, such as deli meats.<br><br>*Condiments, seasonings and spreads.* Herbs, spices, flavored vinegars, salsas and olive oil can add zest to your meals without the salt overload. Choose low- or reduced-sodium versions of condiments.<br><br>*Mayo Clinic* | *Standard DASH diet.* You can consume up to 2,300 milligrams (mg) of sodium a day.<br><br>*Lower sodium DASH diet.* You can consume up to 1,500 mg of sodium a day.<br><br>*Fats* – not heart healthy Saturated fats, including coconut oil, palm oil, and foods containing them.<br><br>*Trans fats /* partially hydrogenated fats and foods containing them – these include many pastries, cookies, and snack crackers, which either contain trans fats or have replaced them with coconut oil or palm oil. Limit fats high in omega-6 fatty acids, such as corn oil, soybean oil (often called vegetable oil), and safflower oil. You can have butter rarely and in small amounts – choose it for special meals for its flavor.<br><br>*Sugary foods* Sugar, honey, agave, molasses, maple syrup, and other sugars Baked goods and pastries. Soda with sugar Candies etc. Energy bars Any other sugary foods<br><br>*Chewfo* | *Rinse it off.* Rinse canned foods, such as tuna, beans, and vegetables, before using to wash away some excess salt.<br><br>*Beware of broth.* Sauté onions, mushrooms or other vegetables in water or a little low-sodium broth. But because even low-sodium broth can add lots of unnecessary sodium, sometimes a healthy oil may be the best option.<br><br>*Make lower fat substitutions.* Use lower fat dairy products, such as reduced-fat cream cheese and fat-free sour cream, instead of their higher fat counterparts.<br><br>*Cut back on meat.* Prepare stews and casseroles with only two-thirds of the meat the recipe calls for, adding extra vegetables, brown rice, tofu, bulgur or whole-wheat pasta instead.<br><br>Caffeine<br><br>*Mayo Clinic* | Avoid caffeine containing medications such as Anacin |

# Cardiac References

## CDC – Center for Disease Control and Prevention

**Other Conditions -** *https://www.cdc.gov/heartdisease/other_conditions.htm*

**Aortic Aneurysm.** *https://www.cdc.gov/dhdsp/data_statistics/fact_sheets/fs_aortic_aneurysm.htm*

**A-fib -** *https://www.cdc.gov/dhdsp/data_statistics/fact_sheets/fs_atrial_fibrillation.htm*

**Blood Pressure (Hypertension)** *https://www.cdc.gov/dhdsp/data_statistics/fact_sheets/fs_bloodpressure.htm*

**Cardiomyopathy -** *https://www.cdc.gov/heartdisease/cardiomyopathy.htm*

**Cholesterol** https://www.cdc.gov/cholesterol/about.htm

**Heart Disease** *https://www.cdc.gov/heartdisease/coronary_ad.htm*

**Heart Failure -** *https://www.cdc.gov/dhdsp/data_statistics/fact_sheets/fs_heart_failure.htm*

**Stroke -** https://www.cdc.gov/stroke/about.htm

## NIH – National Heart, Blood and Lung Institute

**Atherosclerosis -** *https://www.nhlbi.nih.gov/health-topics/atherosclerosis*

**Coronary Heart Disease** - *https://www.nhlbi.nih.gov/health-topics/coronary-heart-disease*

**Heart Attack -** *https://www.nhlbi.nih.gov/health-topics/heart-attack*

**Heart Failure -** *https://www.nhlbi.nih.gov/health-topics/heart-failure*

**Heart-healthy eating -** *https://www.nhlbi.nih.gov/node/24044*

**Heart Murmur -** *https://www.nhlbi.nih.gov/health-topics/heart-murmur*

**Hypotension (Blood Pressure) -** *https://www.nhlbi.nih.gov/health-topics/hypotension*

**Pacemakers -** *https://www.nhlbi.nih.gov/health-topics/pacemakers*

**PAD -** *https://www.nhlbi.nih.gov/health-topics/peripheral-artery-disease*

**Palpitations -** *https://www.nhlbi.nih.gov/health-topics/heart-palpitations*

**Physical Activity and Your Heart -** *https://www.nhlbi.nih.gov/health-topics/physical-activity-and-your-heart*

**Stroke -** *https://www.nhlbi.nih.gov/health-topics/stroke*

**Triglycerides -** *https://www.nhlbi.nih.gov/health-topics/high-blood-triglycerides*

**AUSmed -** *Chronic Heart Failure and Exercise: to Exercise, or Not to Exercise?*
*https://www.ausmed.com/articles/chronic-heart-failure-and-exercise/*

**Cardiomyopathy UK –** *Exercise -* *https://www.cardiomyopathy.org/physical-health/exercise*

**Cinahl Information Systems -** *Peripheral Artery Disease and Exercise* - *https://www.ebscohost.com/assets-sample-content/RRC_Peripheral-Artery-Disease-and-Exercise.pdf*

**Cleveland Clinic -** *Exercise & Activity After a Heart Attack -*
*https://my.clevelandclinic.org/departments/heart/patient-education/recovery-care/interventional-procedures/exercise-activity*

**Doctor's Handbook** *CHF* - https://exerciserx.cheu.gov.hk/files/DoctorsHanbook_ch8.pdf

**E-Pain Assist -** *What Are The Types Of Exercise A Patient With Aortic Aneurysm Should Go For?*
*https://www.epainassist.com/abdominal-pain/aorta/can-you-exercise-if-you-have-an-aortic-aneurysm*

**Everyday Health (EH) -** *8 Exercise Safety Tips for Atrial Fibrillation*
*https://www.everydayhealth.com/hs/atrial-fibrillation-and-stroke/A-fib-exercise-safety-tips/*

**Harvard Medical Publishing** *The Many Ways Exercise Helps Your Heart*
*https://www.health.harvard.edu/heart-health/the-many-ways-exercise-helps-your-heart*

**HealthLine -** *Exercising When You Have Atrial Fibrillation*
*https://www.healthline.com/health/atrial-fibrillation-exercise#effects-of-A-fib-on-exercise*

**HealthLine -** *Implantable Cardioverter Defibrillator (ICD) -*
*https://www.healthline.com/health/implantable-cardioverter-defibrillator*

**Heart Online:** *Exercise response to cardiac medications*    *www.heartonline.org.au/resources*

**LiveStrong -** *Exercise With an Abdominal Aortic Aneurysm -*
*https://www.livestrong.com/article/1013080-livestrongs-future-food-chef-dinner-chef-tal-ronnen-impossible-burger/*

**LiveStrong -** *Heart Arrhythmia & Exercise - https://www.livestrong.com/article/455247-heart-arrhythmia-exercise/*

**LiveStrong -** *Exercises With a Pacemake*r *- https://www.livestrong.com/article/274368-exercises-with-a-pacemaker/*

**Living with Atrial Fibrillation -** *Can I Exercise with Atrial Fibrillation?*
*http://www.livingwithatrialfibrillation.com/2402/exercise-with-atrial-fibrillation/*

**MedScape :** *Angina - Specific Exercise Precautions - Exercising With Angina: Prescription for Health*
*https://www.medscape.com/viewarticle/719400*

**National Stroke Association -** *Hope, A Stroke Recovery Guide*
*http://www.stroke.org/stroke-resources/library/hope-stroke-recovery-guide OR*file:///D:/Documents/Documents/Cardiac/HOPEGuide_2016_FINAL_online.pdf

**Stroke Foundation -** *Mobility And Exercise After Stroke Fact Sheet*
*https://strokefoundation.org.au/About-Stroke/Help-after-stroke/Stroke-resources-and-fact-sheets/Mobility-and-exercise-after-stroke-fact-sheet*

## *Quick Summary* this Section

**Safety First**
- Benefits / Before Starting a Routine
- Averages, Body Temperature
- Respiration, Blood Pressure, Heart Rate
- How to Monitor Intensity of Heart Rate
- Temperature – Heat and Cold
- Dehydration; Altitude

**Components of a Conditioning Program**
- Warm up/cool down
- Duration, Frequency, Intensity & Movement Patterns
- Breathing – Diaphragmatic, Pursed lip and with Exercise
- Equipment That May be Needed

**Self-Tests**:
- Prior to starting program

**Exercise Worksheets:**
- Exercises below with:
  - Exercise name and number for section
    - Reps, Sets, How many times a day and how long a stretch should be held (Ex. 20 seconds)

| EXERCISE<br>Flexibility (Stretching) | EXERCISE NUMBER | PAGE | REPS | SETS | X DAY | HOLD |
|---|---|---|---|---|---|---|
| PRAYER STRETCH and LATERAL | 53 | | | | | |

**Exercises:**
- Myofascial release
- Flexibility / Stretches / ROM
- Core / Abdominal
- Strengthening - Upper and Lower Extremity
- Balance > Lower Extremity Standing Exercises
- Agility
- Endurance/Aerobic Capacity
- Calories
- Worksheet with room for notes under each section

| EXERCISE<br>Core / Stability / Balance | EXERCISE NUMBER | NOTES |
|---|---|---|
| PRONE BALL | 27 | |

**References**

# PHYSICAL AND PSYCHOLOGICAL BENEFITS OF KEEPING PHYSICALLY FIT

- Contributes positively to maintaining a healthy weight, building and maintaining healthy bone density, muscle strength, joint mobility, reducing surgical risks, and strengthening the immune system.
- Helps to prevent or treat serious and life-threatening chronic conditions such as high blood pressure, obesity, heart disease, Type 2 diabetes, insomnia, and depression.
- Endurance exercise before meals lowers blood glucose more than the same exercise after meals.
- It also improves mental health, helps prevent depression, helps to promote or maintain positive self-esteem, and can even augment an individual's sex appeal or body image.

*(Physical Exercise - Wikipedia)*

# Before starting a routine here are some factors to consider

| AGE | Men over 45 and women over 55 should have medical evaluation before starting a vigorous exercise program. If you will be participating in low to moderate exercise, it is suggested that those with, or have signs and symptoms of cardiopulmonary disease, set up a medical evaluation. |
|---|---|
| **MEDICAL AND PHYSICAL CONDITION** | It is very important for you to be aware of any medical or physical problems that may impede your performance. **If you have any of the following issues, please see a medical doctor and/or physical therapist to address issues before starting an exercise program:**<br>• Cardiac issues<br>• Pulmonary issues<br>• Arthritis<br>• Joint pain<br>• Back pain<br>• Diabetes<br>• Acute or Chronic issues, such as, but not limited to, Parkinson's, Stroke, Autoimmune Diseases, Metabolic Disease or Orthopedic disorders/joint replacements. |

# VITAL SIGN AVERAGES

### Adult (resting)

| | |
|---|---|
| **Body Temperature** | 98.6 Fahrenheit under tongue. |
| **Respiration** | 12-20 breaths per minute |
| **Blood Pressure**<br>Systolic/Diastolic | 120/80.<br>Systolic is when the heart pumps blood to the body / Diastolic is blood that remains in arteries when the heart relaxes.<br>*Pre-hypertension*: 120-139/80-89.<br>*Hypertension:*<br>    Stage I 140-159/90-99<br>    Stage II over 160/100 |
| **Resting pulse** | **Men:** 70 beats per minute.<br>**Women:** 75 beats per minute. |

# HOW to MONITOR EXERCISE INTENSITY

### Ways to monitor heart rate (HR):

| | |
|---|---|
| **Talk Test Method** | This is a simple, subjective method for the beginner to determine your comfort zone while exercising. Are you able to breathe and talk comfortably throughout the workout without gasping for air? If not, reduce your activity level, catch your breath, and resume at a slower pace. |
| **Heart Rate monitor or Watch** | This is a device you wear on your wrist or chest, which allows you to measure your heart rate in real time. These devices range in price at about $50.00 for just a basic HR monitor or higher with other bells and whistles. Some of the popular manufacturers are Fitbit, Apple Watch, Garmin and Samsung Galaxy among others. (See *Target Heart Rate*) |
| **Rate of Perceived Exertion** | This method was designed by Dr. Gunnar Borg and is often called the Borg Scale (revised). It rates what you feel your level of exertion is from a scale of 1-10, one being at rest and ten at maximal exertion. A rate of 5-7 is recommended, somewhere between somewhat hard and very hard. Like the talk test method, this is subjective and should be used with HR monitoring. |
| **Training Heart Rate** | Measuring Heart Rate: Place your first and second finger over the pulse site and gently apply pressure. Palpate the number of beats for a full minute or 30 sec x 2, 15 sec x 4 or 6 sec x 10. If you have in irregular heartbeat, it is suggested counting the full 60 seconds. Do not use the thumb, as this has its own pulse. |
| | Take your pulse after you've been exercising for at least five minutes. An easy way to check your pulse without interrupting your workout too much is to take a quick 6-second count and then multiply that number by 10 to get your heart rate in beats per minute (BPM). Make sure your pulse is within your target heart rate zone (*see below*). You can then increase or decrease your intensity based on your heart rate. You can also wear a heart rate monitor.<br><br>Radial: Wrist following line from base of thumb.　　Carotid: Side of larynx. |
| **Target heart rate range (THR)** | **Beginner or low fitness level**: 50-60%<br>**Intermediate or average fitness level:** 60-70%<br>**Advanced or high fitness level:** 75-85% |
| ***Percent of maximal heart rate*** | 220 - Age = predicted maximum heart rate (HR). To get the desired exercise intensity, multiply the predicted maximal HR by the percentage. For example, a woman who is 40 years old of Intermediate fitness level would use the following equation at a 70% target heart rate:<br>220 – 40 (age) =180 predicted maximal HR.<br>180 x 0.70 (THR) = 126 BPM - desired exercise HR. |
| ***Karvonen Formula*** | Percentage of Heart-rate reserve. This formula factors in the resting HR as well, which will make the target heart rate higher than just the percentage of maximal heart rate. To figure this out, take the predicted maximal heart rate as above with a resting HR prior to exercise.<br><br>Maximal HR – resting heart rate (RHR) = heart rate reserve; multiply by intensity + RHR + Target HR. See example under Percentage of maximal HR. Rest heart rate = 80.<br>220 – 40 (age) =180 (as above) – 80 (RHR) = 100 x 0.70 (THR) = 70 + 80 = 150 Target HR. |

# TEMPERATURE – HEAT and COLD

## HEAT

Avoid exercise in the hottest part of the day, as well as in humid weather. People need to sweat to regulate internal body temperature and must evaporate to dissipate heat. During hot, humid weather, sweat cannot evaporate, and therefore cannot cool the body down. It is also important to drink plenty of cool water during exercise, about 7-10 oz. every 10-20 minutes during exercise (see *Dehydration*).

| | |
|---|---|
| **Heat cramps:** | • Severe cramps that begin in hands, feet or calves<br>• Hard, tense muscles |
| **Heat exhaustion:**<br>Requires immediate medical attention, although not usually life threatening | • Fatigue<br>• Nausea<br>• Headache<br>• Excessive thirst<br>• Muscle aches and cramps<br>• Confusion or anxiety<br>• Weakness<br>• Severe sweats that can be accompanied by cold, clammy skin<br>• Slow heartbeat (decreased pulse rate)<br>• Dizziness or fainting<br>• Agitation |
| **Heat Stroke:**<br>Can occur suddenly, with or without warning from heat exhaustion. Obtain immediate medical attention, as this can be *fatal* | • Nausea and vomiting<br>• Headache<br>• Increased body temperature, but DECREASED sweating.<br>• Hot, flushed, DRY skin<br>• Dizziness<br>• Fatigue<br>• Rapid heart rate<br>• Shortness of breath<br>• Decreased urination or may have blood in the urine.<br>• Confusion or loss of consciousness<br>• Convulsions |

# COLD

It is just as important to drink plenty of water when exercising in the cold weather secondary to increased urine production. Be sure to dress in layers to help self-regulate body temperature. This simply involves taking off or putting back on clothing as dictated by the changing weather conditions. Choose clothing that will keep moisture out and away from the skin, such as Gortex® brand. Clothing that stays wet because of sweat will decrease your body temperature.

| | |
|---|---|
| **Hypothermia-Mild:**<br>A body temperature that is below normal. People with hypothermia are usually not aware of their condition due to confusion or being overly focused on their current activity. Hypothermia may or may not include shivering in the early stages | • Confusion<br>• Lack of coordination<br>• Fatigue<br>• Nausea or vomiting<br>• Dizziness |
| **Hypothermia** | • Shivering<br>• Slurred speech<br>• Mumbling<br>• Clumsiness<br>• Difficulty speaking<br>• Stumbling<br>• Poor decision making<br>• Drowsiness<br>• Weak pulse<br>• Shallow breathing<br>• Progressive loss of consciousness |

# DEHYDRATION

Excessive loss of body fluid (which can include water and solutes, usually sodium or electrolytes). It is also important to drink plenty of cool water during exercise, about 7-10 oz. every 10-20 minutes during exercise. During exercise, sports drinks may be necessary to keep an electrolyte balance as well.

| | |
|---|---|
| **Dehydration-Mild:** About 2% of water depletion | • Thirst<br>• Decreased urine volume<br>• Abnormally dark urine<br>• Unexplained tiredness<br>• Irritability<br>• Lack of tears when crying<br>• Headache<br>• Dry mouth<br>• Dizziness when standing due to orthostatic hypotension<br>• May cause insomnia. |
| **Moderate:** About 5% -6% of water depletion | • Grogginess or sleepiness<br>• Headache<br>• Nausea<br>• May feel tingling in limbs (parenthesis) |
| **Severe:** About 10% -15% of water depletion | • Muscles may become spastic<br>• Skin may shrivel and wrinkle (decreased skin turgor)<br>• Vision may dim<br>• Urination will be greatly reduced and may become painful<br>• Delirium may begin. |
| **Over 15% of water depletion** | • Usually, fatal. |

# COMPONENTS OF A CONDITIONING PROGRAM

## WARM UP and COOL DOWN

**Warming up and cooling down are very important parts of the exercise routine. There are physical and psychological benefits to both these components that can be as simple as a slow walk before and after your exercise program.**

| Benefits of warming up | Benefits of cooling down |
|---|---|
| • Increases the temperature in the muscles, which increases the speed of contraction and relaxation.<br>• Reduces premature lactic acid build up and fatigue during high level exercises.<br>• Increases speed of nerve impulse conduction.<br>• Increases elasticity of connective tissues<br>• Increases muscle metabolism and oxygen consumption that enhances aerobic performance.<br>• Alert for potential muscle injury that may arise during higher intensities.<br>• Increases endorphins.<br>• Allows the heart rate to get to a workable rate for beginning exercise.<br>• Increases production of synovial fluid located between the joints to reduce friction.<br>• Psychological warm up to mentally focus on training and competition. | • Prevents venous blood pooling at the extremities, which reduces chance of dizziness or fainting.<br>• Reduces the potential for Delayed Onset Muscle Soreness (DOMS).<br>• Aids in removing waste products in muscles, such as lactic acid.<br>• Reduces the level of adrenaline and other exercise hormones in the blood to lower the chance of post-exercise disturbances in cardiac rhythm.<br>• Allows the heart to return back safely to resting rate. |

### Start out every routine with a warmup first. Here are some suggestions

- Walking or outside
- Running up and down some stairs
- Jumping jacks
- Running in place
- Dynamic stretching

**Equipment**

- Treadmill
- Stationary or Recumbent bike
- Stair climber or Elliptical
- Mini trampoline

# Duration, Frequency, Intensity and Movement Patterns

| | |
|---|---|
| **Intensity:**<br><br>How *much* mental and phys  a  l *effort* it takes to sustain an activity. | This can be done using the target heart rate range THR (optimum exercise intensity levels through beats per minute, talk test or rate of perceived exertion. |
| **Duration:**<br><br>How *long* the training lasts. | The higher the intensity, the shorter the duration.  The American College of Sports Medicine guidelines recommends all healthy adults aged 18–65 y  should participate in moderate intensity aerobic physical activity for a minimum of 30 min on five days per week, or vigorous intensity aerobic activity for a minimum of 20 min on three days per week. |
| **Frequency:**<br><br>How *often* the training occurs. | Training should be performed at least every other day or three days a week.  Cardiac/aerobic conditioning can be done daily, although you may want to a ry exercises.<br>Regarding strength training, it is important to give each mus  e group 48 hours to recover.  Alternate upper and lower body with isolated abdomen/core exercises every other day.  For those working out several days a week, find a schedule that works for you as long as you give each muscle group 48 hours of recovery time. |
| **Movement Patterns and Examples**<br><br>Basic movements that help to increase overall body strengthening | • Bend and Lift:  Squats, Dead Lifts and Leg presses<br>  o Picking up item off floor<br>• Single Leg: Step ups, Single leg s ane , Lunges<br>  o Walking up steps<br>• Push:  Shoulder press, Bench pres   Push up<br>  o Pushing Shopping cart or Lawn mower<br>• Pull: Lat pull downs, Seated rows<br>  o Vacuuming, Raking<br>• Rotational<br>  o Shoveling snow |

## Diaphragmatic Breathing

• Lie either on your back with your knees bent or sit up
• Inhale through your nose; as you do so, allow your stomach to rise. Limit movement in your chest. Attempt to push your bottom ribs out to the side as you breathe in.
• Exhale through your mouth; as you do so, allow your stomach to fall.  Limit movement in your chest.
• Repeat for at least 10 cycles.

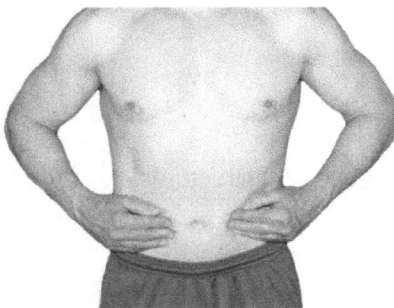

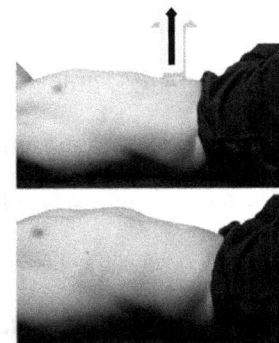

## Pursed Lip Breathing

(PLB) is a breathing technique that consists of inhaling through the nose with the mouth closed and then exhaling through tightly pressed (pursed) lips.  This technique is frequently in those with cardiac or respiratory issues.      *"Smell the Roses then Blow Out the Candle"*.

## Breathing with Exercise

Exhale on the exertion. For example, exhale when you are lying on your back and pushing a weight up or when bending your arm doing a bicep curl,.  Inhale as you bring the weight slowly to your b es  or when you straighten your arm with a bicep curl..

# ANATOMY
## ANATOMICAL POSITIONS and PLANES

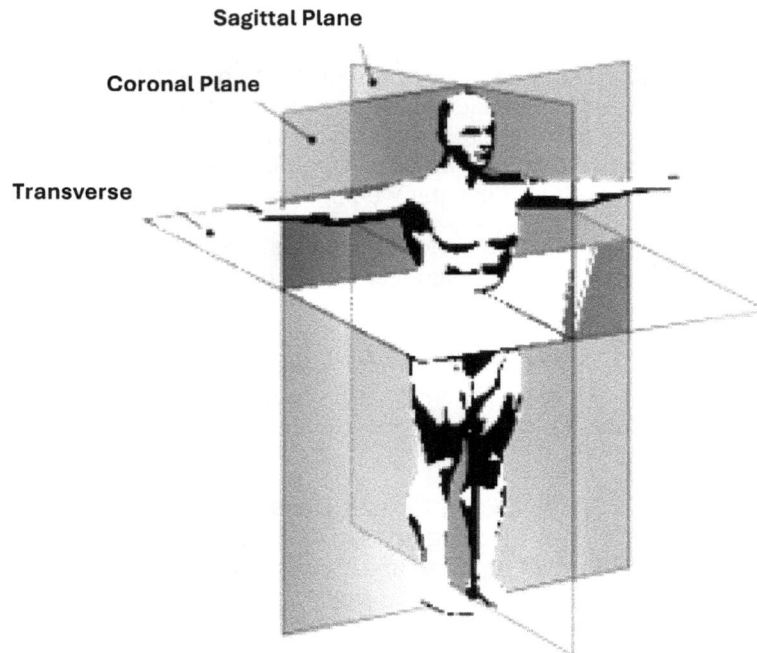

**Anterior** – Towards the front of the body.

**Posterior** – Towards the back of the body.

**Distal** – Away from the body or any point of reference, or from the point of attachment or origin.

**Proximal** – Closer to the body or any point of reference, or to the point of attachment or origin.

**Medial** – Situated towards the midline of the body.

**Lateral** – Position farther from the midline of the body.

**Inferior** – Away from the head or lower surface of a structure.

**Superior** – Towards the head or situated above.

**Transverse /Axial / Horizontal plane** is parallel to the ground, which separates the superior from the inferior or the head from the feet.

**Coronal / Frontal/Frontal plane** is perpendicular to the ground, which separates the anterior from the posterior or the front from the back

**Sagittal / Lateral plane** is a Y-Z plane, perpendicular to the ground, which separates left from right.

**Upper Extremity (UE):** Shoulders, Chest, Arms, Hands, etc

**Lower Extremity (LE):** Hips, Legs, Ankle Foot , etc

# ANATOMICAL DIRECTIONS

**Range of Motion (ROM):** The distance and direction a joint can move between the flexed and extended position (*see flexion and extension below*). This can also be the act of attempting to increase the distance through therapeutic exercise and/or stretching for physiological gain.

**Flexion** - Bending movement that decreases the angle between two parts. Bending the knee or elbow are examples of flexion. Flexion of the hip or shoulder moves the limb forward (towards the front of the body).

**Extension** - The opposite of flexion; a straightening movement that increases the angle between body parts. The knees are extended when standing up. When straightening the arm, the elbow is extended. Extension of the hip or shoulder moves the limb backward (towards the back of the body).

**Hyperextension** – Extending the joint beyond extension.

**Abduction** - A lateral movement that pulls a structure or part away from the midline of the body. Raising the arms to the sides is an example of abduction.

**Adduction** - A medial movement that pulls a structure or part towards the midline of the body, or towards the midline of a limb. Dropping the arms to the sides, or bringing the knees together, are examples of adduction.

**Internal rotation** (or *medial rotation*). Inward rotary movement around the axis of the bone. Internal rotation of the shoulder or hip would point the toes or the flexed forearm inwards (towards the midline).

**External rotation** (or *lateral rotation*). External rotary movement around the axis of the bone. It would turn the toes or the flexed forearm outwards (away from the midline).

**Elevation** - Movement in a superior direction. Shrugging or bringing the shoulders up is an example of elevation.

**Depression** - Movement in an inferior direction, the opposite of elevation. Pushing the shoulders down is an example of depression.

**Pronation** - Internal rotation the hand or foot to face downward or posterior. Pronating the foot is a combination of eversion and abduction.

**Supination** - External rotation of the hand or foot to face upward or anterior. Raising the inside or medial margin of the foot.

**Dorsiflexion** – Movement at the ankle of the foot superiorly towards the shin. The up position of tapping the foot.

**Plantarflexion** – Movement at the ankle of the foot inferiorly away from the shin. Pointing the foot downward.

**Eversion** – Moving the sole of the foot away from the median plane or outward.

**Inversion** - Moving the sole of the foot towards the median plane or inward.

**Ipsilateral** – Same side of the body

**Contralateral** – Opposite side of the body

# MUSCLES

*Grey's Anatomy*

## ANTERIOR

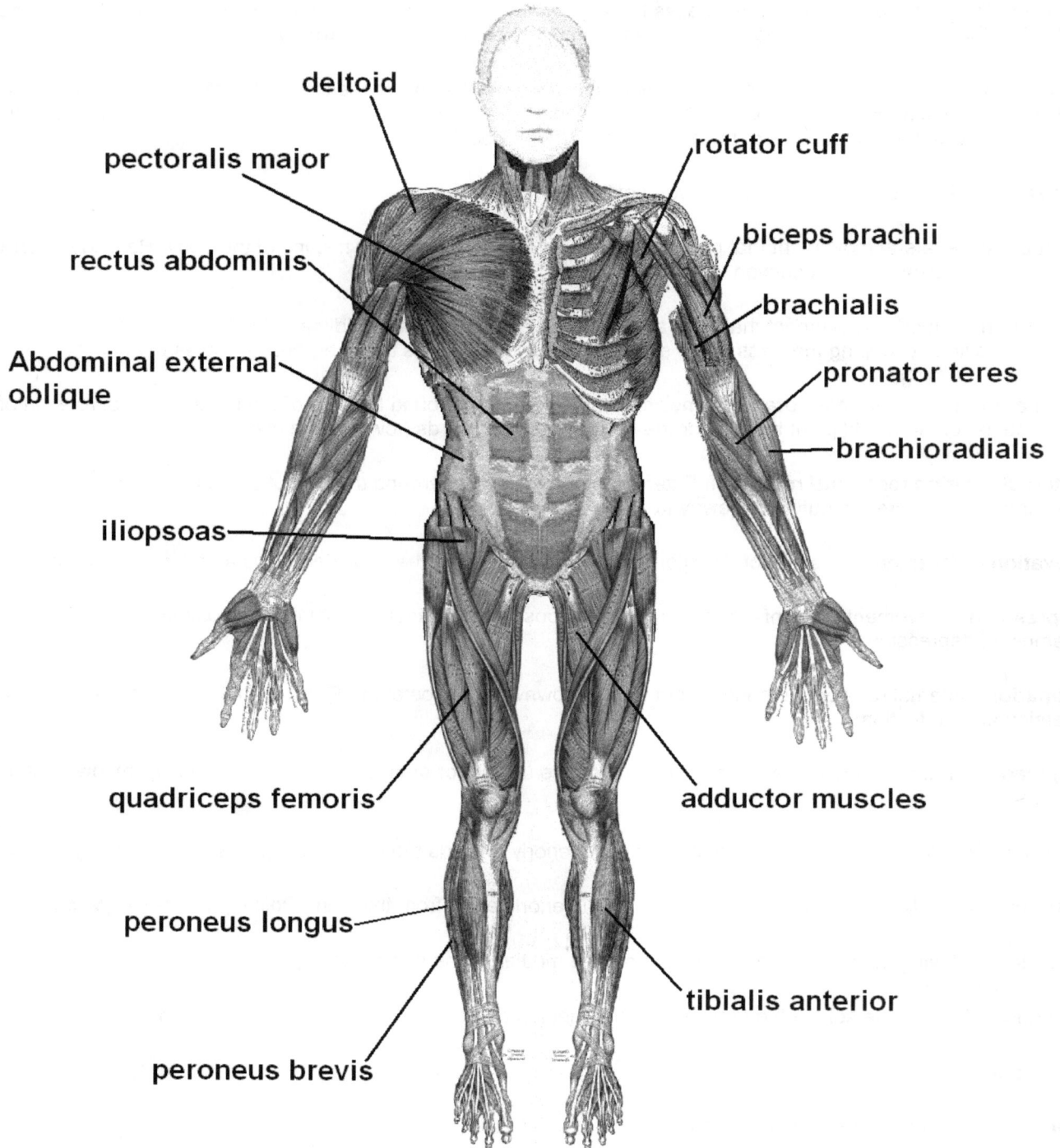

deltoid

pectoralis major

rectus abdominis

Abdominal external oblique

iliopsoas

quadriceps femoris

peroneus longus

peroneus brevis

rotator cuff

biceps brachii

brachialis

pronator teres

brachioradialis

adductor muscles

tibialis anterior

| Muscle Name (AKA) | Joint Action |
|---|---|
| Pectoralis major | Shoulder flexion, adduction, internal rotation |
| Deltoid (anterior) | Shoulder abduction, flexion, internal rotation |
| Rotator cuff (SITS) Supraspinatus Infraspinatus Teres minor Subscapularis | Shoulder: Supraspinatus: Abduction Infraspinatus: External rotation Teres minor: External rotation Subscapularis: Internal rotation |
| Biceps brachii | Elbow flexion; Forearm supination |
| Brachialis | Elbow flexion |
| Pronator teres | Elbow flexion; Forearm pronation |
| Brachioradialis | Elbow flexion |
| Tensor fasciae latae | Hip flexion, medial rotation & abduction |
| Gracilis* | Hip adduction & internal rotation;Knee flexion & internal rotation |
| Adductor muscles Adductor magnus, longus & brevis | Hip adduction |
| Tibialis anterior | Ankle dorsiflexion; foot inversion |
| Peroneus brevis | Ankle plantarflexion; Foot eversion |
| Peroneus longus | Ankle plantarflexion; Foot eversion |
| Rectus femoris (quadriceps femoris) | Hip extension (esp. when knee is extended); Knee flexion |
| Vastus medialis | Knee extension (esp. when hip is flexed) |
| Vastus lateralis | Knee extension (esp. when hip is flexed) |
| Sartorius | Hip flexion & external rotation; Knee flexion & internal rotation |
| Pectineus | Hip adduction |
| Iliopsoas, Psosas, Iliacus | Hip flexion & external rotation |
| Abdominal external oblique | Trunk lateral flexion |
| Rectus abdominis | Trunk flexion & lateral flexion |
| Abdominal internal oblique | Trunk lateral flexion |

# MUSCLES

*Grey's Anatomy*

**POSTERIOR**

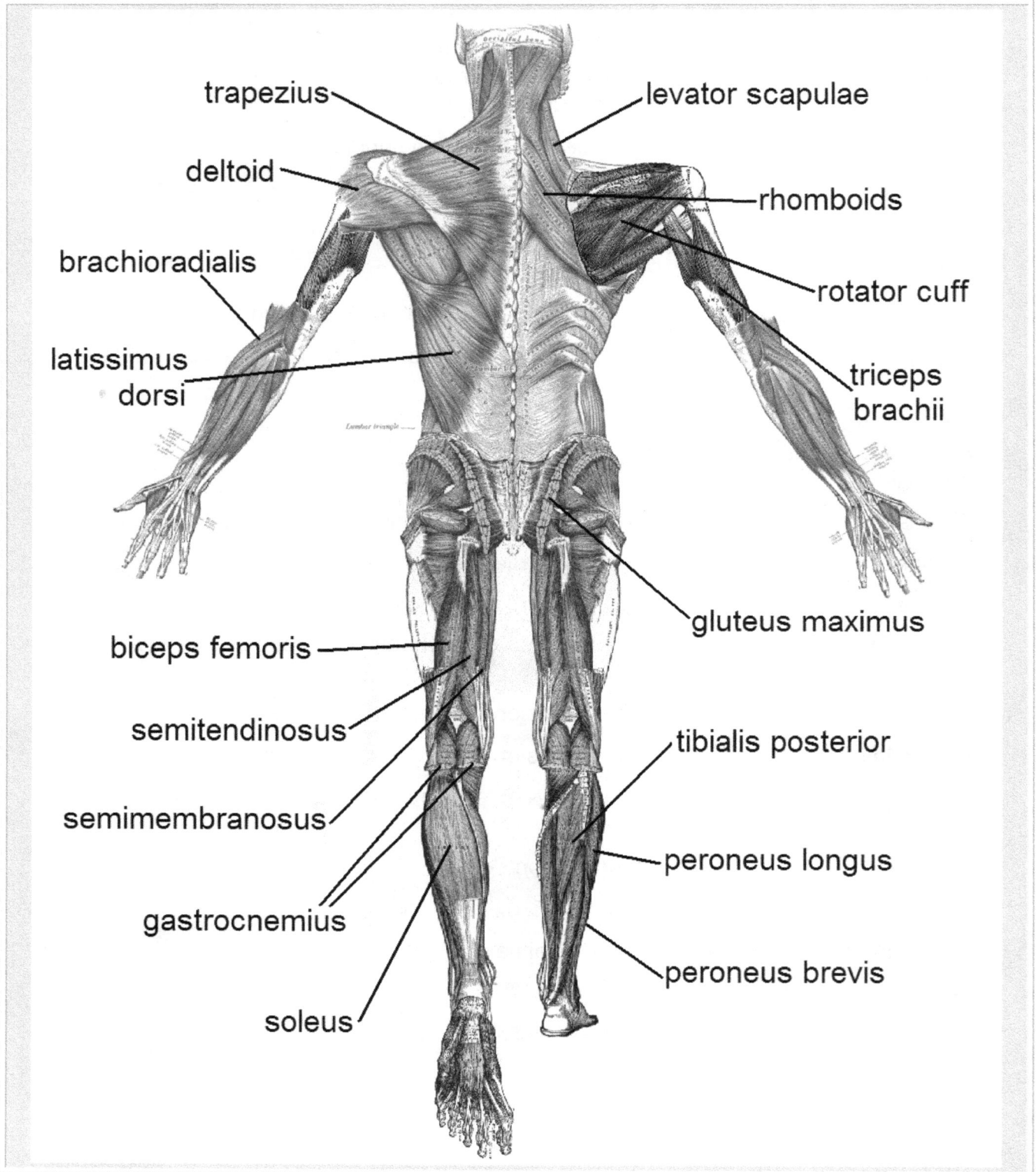

trapezius

levator scapulae

deltoid

rhomboids

brachioradialis

rotator cuff

latissimus dorsi

triceps brachii

biceps femoris

gluteus maximus

semitendinosus

tibialis posterior

semimembranosus

peroneus longus

gastrocnemius

peroneus brevis

soleus

| Muscle Name (AKA) | Joint Action |
|---|---|
| Deltoid (posterior) | Shoulder abduction, extension, external rotation |
| Trapezius | Scapula or Shoulder girdle:, Upper traps: Scapula elevation.<br>Middle traps: Scapula adduction.<br>Lower traps:  Scapula depression |
| Levator scapulae | Scapula elevation |
| Rhomboids | Scapula adduction & elevation |
| Triceps brachii | Elbow extension |
| Gluteus medius | Hip abduction |
| Gluteus maximus | Hip extension & external rotation |
| Tibialis, posterior | Inversion, stabilization, assists with plantarflexion |
| Soleus | Ankle plantarflexion |
| Gastrocnemius | Knee flexion; Ankle plantarflexion |
| Semimembranosus | Hip extension & internal rotation;<br>Knee flexion & internal rotation |
| Semitendinosus | Hip extension & internal rotation; Knee flexion & internal rotation |
| Biceps femoris (long head) | Hip extension & internal rotation;<br>Knee flexion & external rotation |
| Latissimus dorsi | Shoulder extension, adduction, internal rotation |
| Erector  spinae, Longissimus, Spinalis, Iliocostalis | Trunk extension, hyperextension & lateral flexion<br><br>Deep muscle that originate in the posterior iliac crest & sacrum running up the spine and inserts in the transverse process of ribs |
| Pes anserine, Gracilis, Sartorius, Semimembranosus, Semitendinosus | Internal rotation of tibia when knee is flexed |

# SKELETON

## ANTERIOR (FRONT)

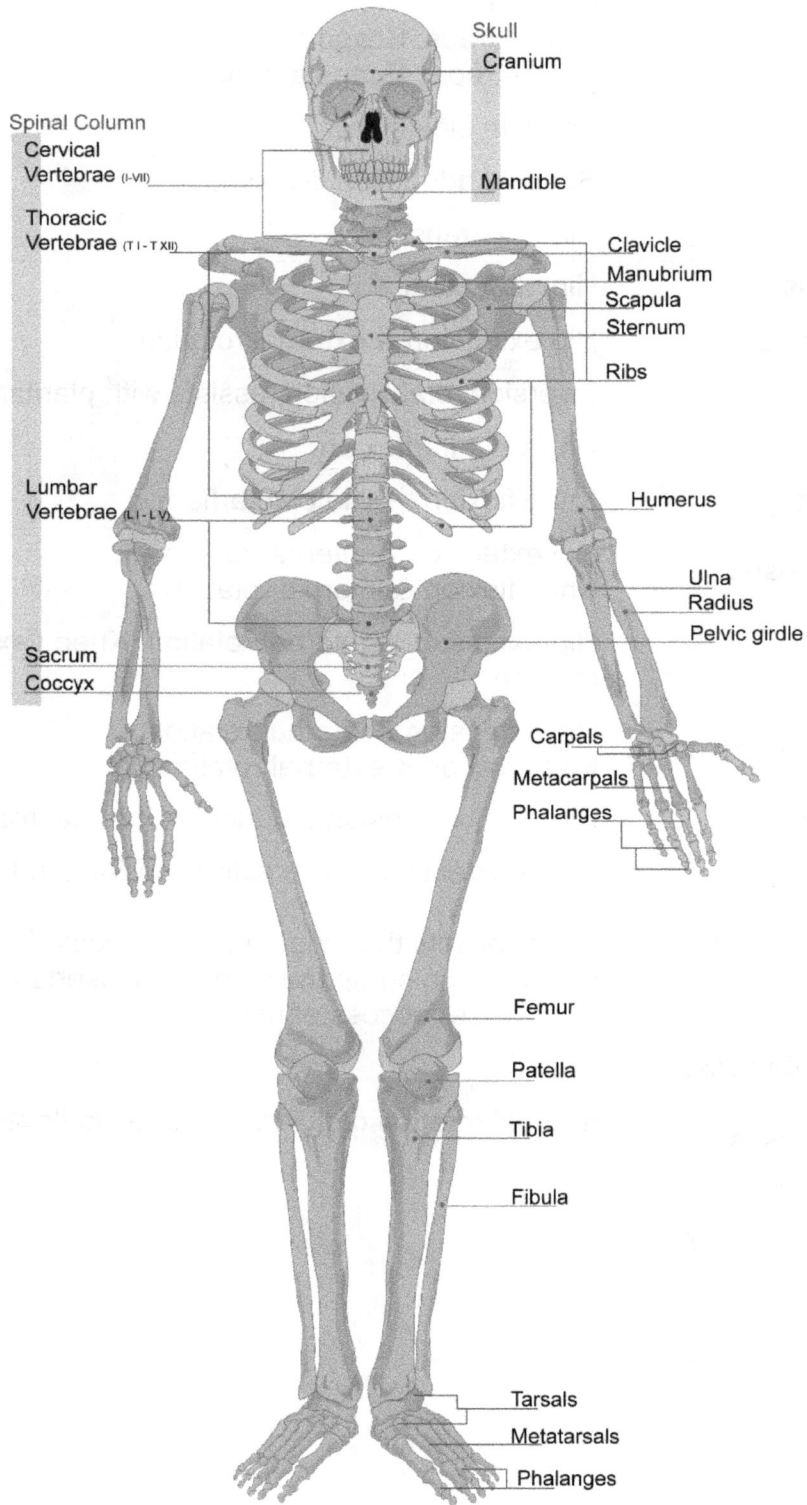

Skull
Cranium

Spinal Column
Cervical
Vertebrae (I-VII)

Thoracic
Vertebrae (T I - T XII)

Mandible

Clavicle
Manubrium
Scapula
Sternum

Ribs

Lumbar
Vertebrae (L I - L V)

Humerus

Ulna
Radius

Pelvic girdle

Sacrum
Coccyx

Carpals

Metacarpals

Phalanges

Femur

Patella

Tibia

Fibula

Tarsals

Metatarsals

Phalanges

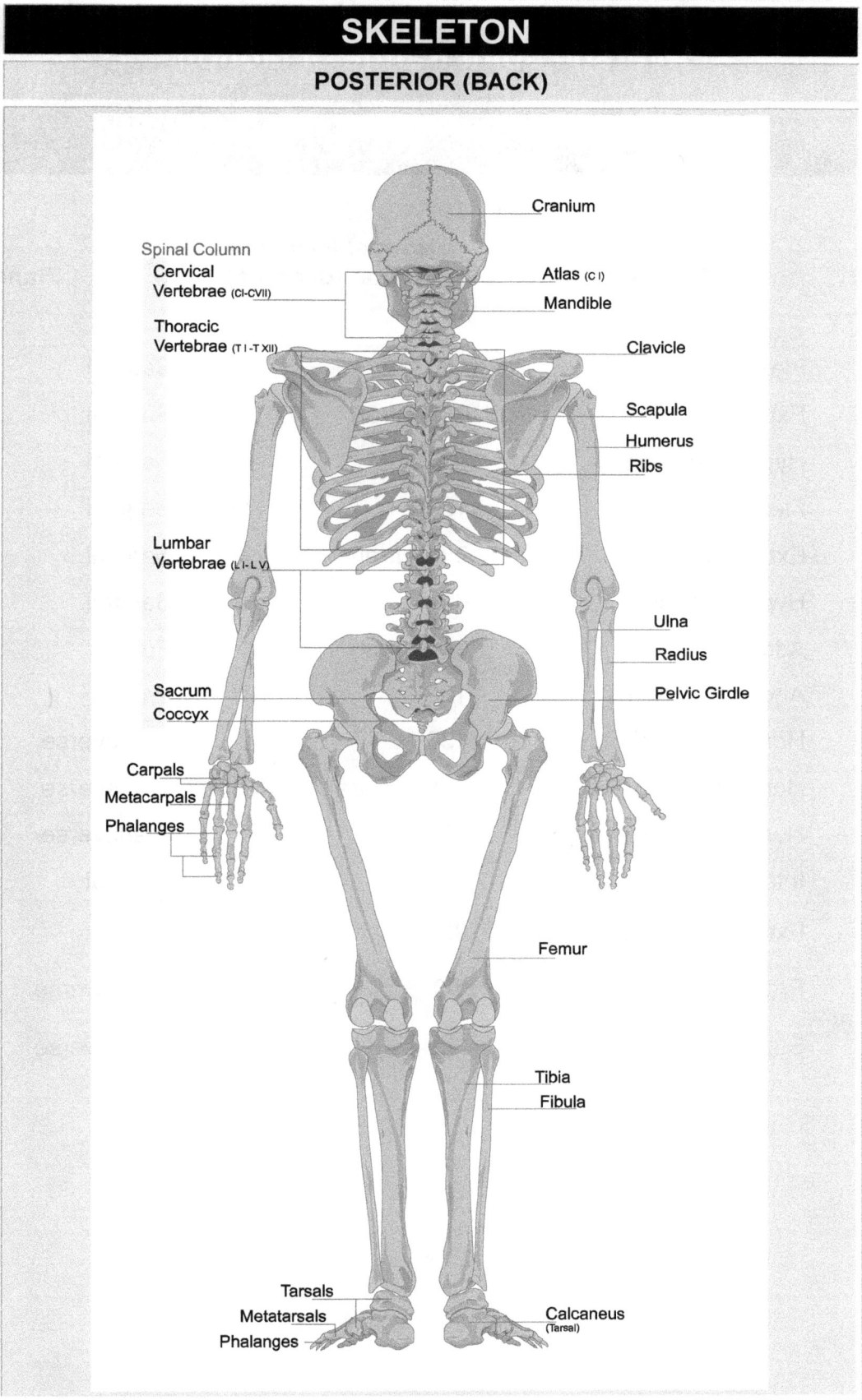

# SKELETON

## POSTERIOR (BACK)

Cranium

Spinal Column

Cervical Vertebrae (CI-CVII)

Atlas (C I)

Mandible

Thoracic Vertebrae (T I -T XII)

Clavicle

Scapula

Humerus

Ribs

Lumbar Vertebrae (L I -L V)

Ulna

Radius

Sacrum

Coccyx

Pelvic Girdle

Carpals

Metacarpals

Phalanges

Femur

Tibia

Fibula

Tarsals

Metatarsals

Phalanges

Calcaneus (Tarsal)

# Average Joint Range of Motion

# Anatomical Positions – Upper Extremity

| Joint<br><br>UPPER EXTREMITY | Movement | Normal Range of Motion (degrees) | Plane |
|---|---|---|---|
| **Elbow** | Flexion | 150 | Sagittal |
| | Extension | 0 (neutral) | Sagittal |
| | Hyperextension | < 10 | Sagittal |
| **Shoulder** | Flexion | 180 | Sagittal |
| | Extension | 0 (neutral) | Sagittal |
| | Hyperextension | 60 | Sagittal |
| | Adduction (Add) | 0 (neutral) | Frontal |
| | Abduction (Abd) | 180 | Frontal |
| | Horizontal Add/Flexion | 130 | Transverse |
| | Horizontal Abd | 0 (to neutral) | Transverse |
| | Horizontal Extension | 45 | Transverse |
| | Internal rotation | 70 | Sagittal |
| | External rotation | 90 | Sagittal |
| **Radioulnar** | Pronation | 90 | Transverse |
| | Supination | 90 | Transverse |

## Average Joint Range of Motion

## Anatomical Positions – Lower Extremity

| Joint<br>LOWER EXTREMITY | Movement | Normal Range of Motion (degrees) | Plane |
|---|---|---|---|
| Knee | Flexion | 135 | Sagittal |
| | Extension | 0 (neutral) | Sagittal |
| | Hyperextension | 10 | Sagittal |
| Hip | Flexion | 120 | Sagittal |
| | Extension | 0 (neutral) | Sagittal |
| | Hyperextension | < 20 | Sagittal |
| | Adduction (Add) | 0 (neutral) | Frontal |
| | Abduction (Abd) | 50 | Frontal |
| | Internal rotation | 40 | Transverse |
| | External rotation | 50 | Transverse |
| Ankle | Dorsiflexion | 20 | Sagittal |
| | Plantarflexion | 50 | Sagittal |

# EQUIPMENT used in this Book.

*Don't buy a lot of equipment before knowing what your goals are.*

| | | |
|---|---|---|
| **Stability / Exercise Ball Bosu**<br><br>These can replace an exercise bench if you do not have the space. It is also used for many of the core strengthening exercises | Should be inflated so that when you sit on it you are at a 90-degree angle. | |

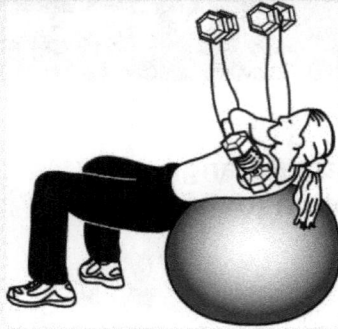

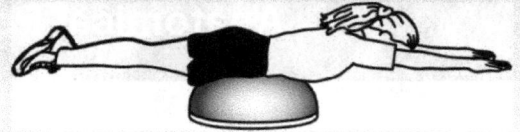

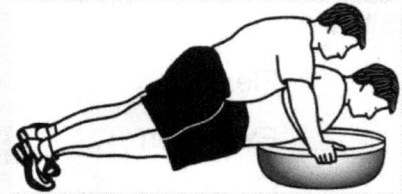

| | | |
|---|---|---|
| **Dumbbells**<br><br>**Kettle Bell** (optional)<br><br>**Dowel with/without weight**<br><br>These will be needed for your strength exercises. See *Strengthening* section on for resistance. | | |

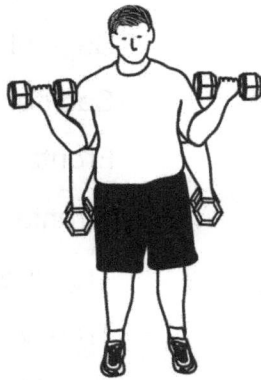

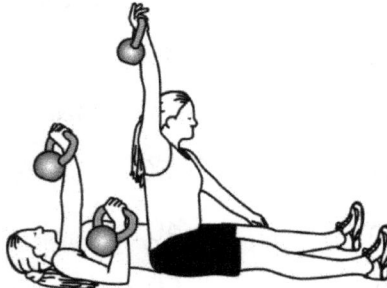

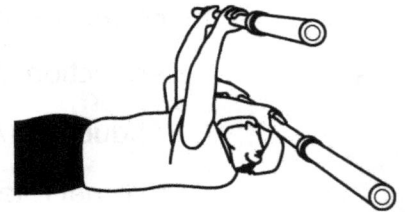

| | |
|---|---|
| **Resistance bands**<br><br>In different weights/ resistance. | |

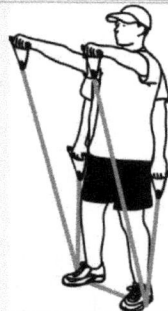

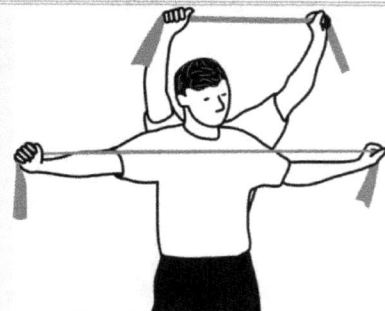

| | | |
|---|---|---|
| **Agility Equipment**<br><br>Cone hurdles, Speed hurdles, Agility ladder/rings/poles, Bosu, Stair step, Jump rope. | | |

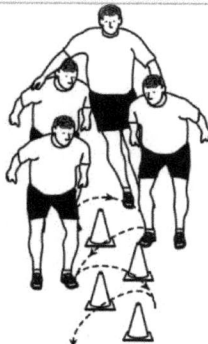

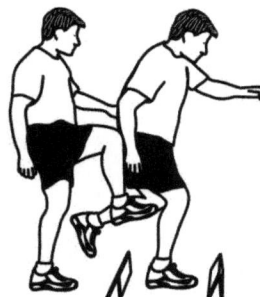

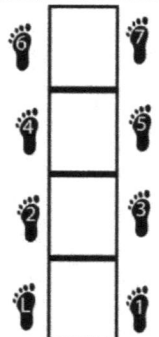

**Balance Equipment**

Can include **Foam rollers** *(also see Myofascial below)*

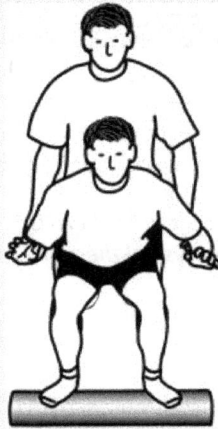

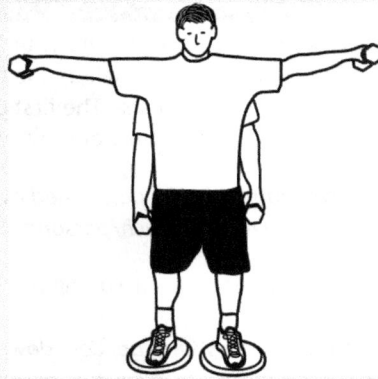

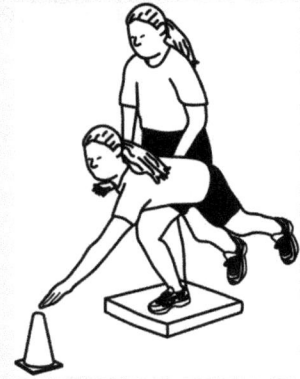

**Balance discs**
**Balance pad**
**Cones**
**Stepper**
**Bosu**

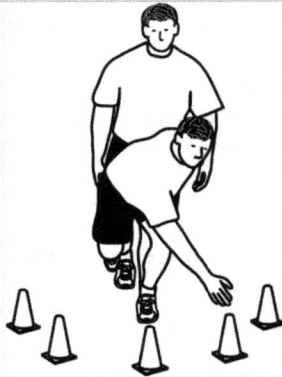

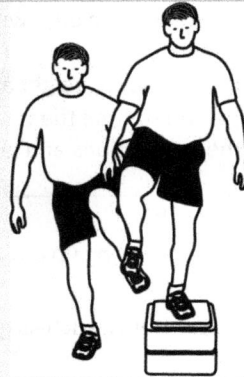

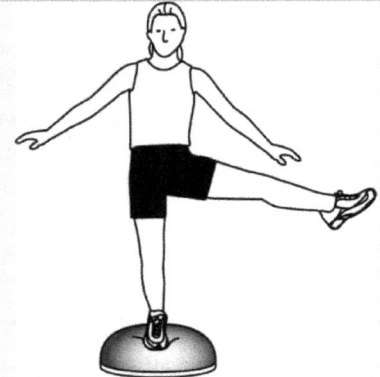

## Exercise Bench (Optional)

The type really depends on what you will use it for. You can get a plain bench just for support (as above you can use a stability ball) or you can get all the bells and whistles. Some have pieces for leg extensions and curls, as well as arm pieces for butterflies. If you do not already have one, I suggest waiting until you start your exercise program and see what you feel you will need to advance.

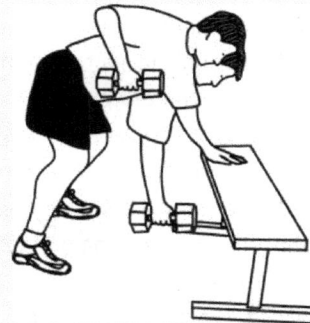

*Examples For Myofascial*

**Massage Ball**

**Foam/Textured Rollers** *(also see balance)*

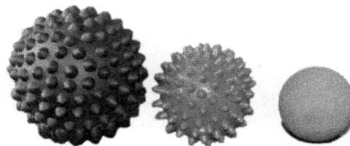

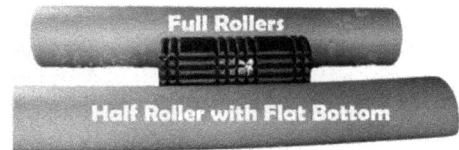

Full Rollers

Half Roller with Flat Bottom

**Not Shown**

- Exercise mat for floor exercises
- Ankle Weights
- Bed, couch or high table/mat
- Chair with/without arms - High or Low

- 10-inch play ball
- Pillow
- Towel roll
- Strap for stretches

# SELF TESTS

Before starting the exercise program, it is a good idea to see where your baseline is. Taking the following tests will help guide you in the level you will need to start, and help progress by retaking the test periodically. *It is suggested to get a partner to help with both timing and safety, especially with balance tests.* The first 6 tests are modified versions starting at age 60 but are great for adults of any age. Tests 7-10 will help determine how quickly you can advance your balance program.

*As with the exercises in this book, these tests should also be performed by those that are otherwise healthy with no chronic or acute ailments OR with supervision of a qualified health coach/personal trainer/physical therapist.*

Tests 1-6 should be conducted in the following order if you are doing them at the same time.

A general warm up should be done prior to tests (*see Warm up/Cool down*).
- Stop immediately if any adverse reactions, such as nausea, dizziness, blurred vision, pain of any kind, chest pain, confusion or loss of muscle control.
- Stay hydrated, and do not proceed with testing on days with high temperature/humidity or any other conditions where you would not normally exercise.
- Practice each test several times before attempting to get an accurate score.
- It is advised that you have a second person to time the tests and make sure you are following proper form. Make sure your partner also understands the precautions and goals of these tests.

1. 30 second chair stand - Lower body strength
   - Needed for stair climbing, walking getting up out of tub/chair/car and reduce the risk of falls
2. 30 second arm curl test – Upper body strength
   - Needed to lift and carry everyday items, such as groceries and toolbox
3. 2-minute step test – Aerobic endurance
   - Needed for activities that require endurance, such as walking distance, grocery shopping and climbing stairs
4. Chair sit and reach – Lower body flexibility
   - Needed for normal gait patterns, correct posture, getting in/out of car/tub
5. Back stretch test – Shoulder flexibility
   - Needed to do various activities, such as combing hair and putting on overhead garments
6. 8 foot get up and go – Agility and dynamic balance
   - Needed for pretty much anything you do that requires getting up and walking, such as go to kitchen, bathroom or answering phone.
7. Narrow stance – Balance progression
8. Staggered stance – Balance progression
9. Tandem stance – Balance progression
10. One leg standing – Balance progression

| TEST AND PURPOSE | PICTURE | EQUIPMENT NEEDED | EXPLANATION | RESULTS |
|---|---|---|---|---|
| **30 Second Chair Stand**<br><br>Assess lower body strength<br><br>*May not want to perform if any chronic pain or back issues.<br>*If you are tall and have had a recent hip replacement skip this or use taller chair. | | Straight back or folding chair (~17 inch height) against wall.<br><br>Stopwatch, wrist watch or clock within view with second hand | *Sit with feet flat on the floor and arms crossed over the chest.<br>*Get up to a full stand and then sit back down.<br>** Start the time – Immediately repeat as many *full stands* as you can in 30 seconds.<br>*If you cannot stand with hands over chest, try pushing off on your thighs or get a chair with arms and push off arms. If using assist, make sure you note this for progression.* | **Normal Range repetitions**<br><br>| Age | Men | Women |<br>|---|---|---|<br>| 60-64 | 14-19 | 12-17 |<br>| 65-69 | 12-18 | 11-16 |<br>| 70-74 | 12-17 | 10-15 |<br>| 75-79 | 11-17 | 10-15 |<br>| 80-84 | 10-15 | 9-14 |<br>| 85-89 | 8-14 | 8-13 |<br>| 90-94 | 7-12 | 4-11 | |

Expanded for clarity:

### 30 Second Chair Stand

| TEST AND PURPOSE | PICTURE | EQUIPMENT NEEDED | EXPLANATION | RESULTS |
|---|---|---|---|---|
| **30 Second Chair Stand**<br><br>Assess lower body strength<br><br>*May not want to perform if any chronic pain or back issues.<br>*If you are tall and have had a recent hip replacement skip this or use taller chair. | | Straight back or folding chair (~17 inch height) against wall.<br><br>Stopwatch, wrist watch or clock within view with second hand | *Sit with feet flat on the floor and arms crossed over the chest.<br>*Get up to a full stand and then sit back down.<br>** Start the time – Immediately repeat as many *full stands* as you can in 30 seconds.<br>*If you cannot stand with hands over chest, try pushing off on your thighs or get a chair with arms and push off arms. If using assist, make sure you note this for progression.* | (see Normal Range repetitions table below) |

**Normal Range repetitions**

| Age | Men | Women |
|---|---|---|
| 60-64 | 14-19 | 12-17 |
| 65-69 | 12-18 | 11-16 |
| 70-74 | 12-17 | 10-15 |
| 75-79 | 11-17 | 10-15 |
| 80-84 | 10-15 | 9-14 |
| 85-89 | 8-14 | 8-13 |
| 90-94 | 7-12 | 4-11 |

### 30 Second Arm Curl Test

| TEST AND PURPOSE | PICTURE | EQUIPMENT NEEDED | EXPLANATION | RESULTS |
|---|---|---|---|---|
| **30 Second Arm Curl Test**<br><br>Upper body strength | | Straight back or folding chair without arms. Can be done in standing.<br><br>Stopwatch or clock within view with second hand<br><br>Women:<br>5 lb dumbbell<br>Men:<br>8 lb dumbbell<br><br>Can use a wrist weight if arthritis and cannot hold a dumbbell | *Sit with feet flat on the floor towards the edge seat towards dominant side.<br>**Start with the arm extended by your side holding dumbbell in the dominant hand.<br>*Bend elbow with palm facing you keeping the upper arm next to the body (elbow pressed into your side).<br>*Return to starting position.<br>*Keep the wrist straight – do not flex or extend the wrist.<br>**Start the time – Immediately repeat as many arm curls as you can in 30 seconds *with proper form.*<br>*If you cannot hold the suggested weight with proper form, use a lighter weight. Make sure you note this for progression.* | (see Normal Range repetitions table below) |

**Normal Range repetitions**

| Age | Men | Women |
|---|---|---|
| 60-64 | 16-22 | 13-19 |
| 65-69 | 15-21 | 12-18 |
| 70-74 | 14-21 | 12-17 |
| 75-79 | 13-19 | 11-17 |
| 80-84 | 13-19 | 10-16 |
| 85-89 | 11-17 | 10-15 |
| 90-94 | 10-14 | 8-13 |

| TEST AND PURPOSE | PICTURE | EQUIPMENT NEEDED | EXPLANATION | RESULTS |
|---|---|---|---|---|
| **2 Minute Step Test**<br><br>Aerobic endurance | | Wall for support and to mark step height.<br><br>Sturdy chair to hold on opposite side if unsteady.<br><br>Stopwatch or clock within view with second hand | \*For accuracy, may need a second person to judge step height and count.<br>\*Step with side next to wall. Bring knee up mid-thigh between the knee and the hip. Mark the wall with tape at this height. This will be your minimum step height.<br>\*Practice marching in place to this step height.<br>\*\*Start the time – Immediately start marching (not jogging) for 2 minutes. Count the number of *full steps* (both legs) that come up to step height. Every time the right knee reaches proper step height; this is counted as one step.<br>*\*If shortness of breath, extreme fatigue or unable to continue to step height, stop test and this is your baseline.*<br>*\* If unable to get to step height, but able to complete 2 minutes. Make sure you note this for progression.*<br>*\*If unsteady, hold onto chair on opposite side for support.* | **Normal Range steps**<br><table><tr><td>Age</td><td>Men</td><td>Women</td></tr><tr><td>60-64</td><td>87-115</td><td>75-107</td></tr><tr><td>65-69</td><td>86-116</td><td>73-107</td></tr><tr><td>70-74</td><td>80-110</td><td>68-101</td></tr><tr><td>75-79</td><td>73-109</td><td>68-100</td></tr><tr><td>80-84</td><td>71-103</td><td>60-90</td></tr><tr><td>85-89</td><td>59-91</td><td>55-85</td></tr><tr><td>90-94</td><td>52-86</td><td>44-72</td></tr></table> |

| TEST AND PURPOSE | PICTURE | EQUIPMENT NEEDED | EXPLANATION | RESULTS |
|---|---|---|---|---|
| **Chair Sit And Reach**<br><br>Lower body flexibility, *primarily hamstrings*<br><br>*Do not do if recent hip replacement or severe osteoporosis.<br><br>*Stretch to discomfort, not pain. | | Chair (~17 inch height). Make sure chair is secure and does not tip forward.<br><br>18 inch ruler or yardstick | *Sit on the edge chair – you should feel the middle of the thigh at the edge of the chair.<br>*Bend one leg with foot flat on floor.<br>*Straighten the target leg in front with heel on the floor and foot flexed up.<br>*Reach forward with one hand over the other and middle fingers even.<br>*Exhale as you bend forward at the hips and reach forward towards or past the toes. Keep the extended knee straight and adjust if it bends.<br>*Practice a few times on both legs to see which one you would prefer for testing. Do two tests and measure as below.<br>**Measure tips of middle fingers to the tip of the shoe (closest to ½ inch).<br>***The midpoint at the toe of the shoe is considered zero (0), and is scored as such if you reach this point.<br>***If the reach is short, score this as a minus (-)<br>***If the reach is past this point, score this as a plus (+) | See table below |

**Normal Range inches**

| Age | Men | Women |
|---|---|---|
| 60-64 | -2.5 +4.0 | -0.5 + 5.0 |
| 65-69 | -3.0 +3.0 | -0.5 + 4.5 |
| 70-74 | -3.0 +3.0 | -1.0 + 4.0 |
| 75-79 | -4.0 +2.0 | -1.5 + 3.5 |
| 80-84 | -5.5 +1.5 | 2.0 + 3.0 |
| 85-89 | -5.5 +0.5 | -2.5 + 2.5 |
| 90-94 | -6.5 -0.5 | -4.5 + 1.0 |

| TEST AND PURPOSE | PICTURE | EQUIPMENT NEEDED | EXPLANATION | RESULTS |
|---|---|---|---|---|
| **Back Stretch Test**<br><br>Shoulder flexibility<br><br>*Do not do if any upper back, shoulder or neck injuries | | 18-inch ruler or yardstick | *Will need second person to measure.<br>*Stand and place the target arm over the same shoulder, palm down with fingers extended. Reach down the middle of the back.<br>*Place the opposite arm around the back, palm up reaching up the middle of the back towards other hand. Try to touch middle fingers together or overlap if possible. *Do not overlap fingers and pull.*<br>*Practice a few times on both arms to see which one you would prefer for testing. Do two tests and measure as below.<br>**Measure the distance between tips of middle fingers or overlap.<br>***If the middle fingers do not touch, score this as a minus (-)<br>***If the middle fingers just touch, score this as a zero (0)<br>***If the middle fingers overlap, score this as a plus (+) | See table below |

**Normal Range inches**

| Age | Men | Women |
|---|---|---|
| 60-64 | -6.5 +0.0 | -3.0 + 1.5 |
| 65-69 | -7.5 -1.0 | -3.5 + 1.5 |
| 70-74 | -8.0 -1.0 | -4.0 + 1.0 |
| 75-79 | -9.0 -2.0 | -5.0 + 0.5 |
| 80-84 | -9.5 -2.0 | -5.5 + 0.0 |
| 85-89 | -9.5 -3.0 | -7.0 -1.0 |
| 90-94 | -10.5 -4.0 | -8.0 -1.0 |

| TEST AND PURPOSE | PICTURE | EQUIPMENT NEEDED | EXPLANATION | RESULTS |
|---|---|---|---|---|
| **8 Foot Get Up And Go**<br><br>Agility and dynamic balance<br><br>*If unsteady, have someone by your side in case you lose your balance. | | Chair against wall (~17-inch height)<br><br>Cone or another marker to walk around<br><br>Stopwatch or clock within view with second hand<br><br>*Put chair against wall and cone 8 feet in front. Measure from front of chair to back of cone (side facing chair).<br><br>8 feet → | *This is done better with a partner watching the clock or a stopwatch.<br>*Sit on chair, back straight, feet flat on floor, one foot slightly in front, torso leaning slightly forward and hands resting on thighs.<br>**Start the time – Immediately get up and walk around the cone (either side) and return to chair. Stopwatch immediately when seated.<br>**Try 2-3x and record the fastest time within 10th /second.<br>*Can use a cane or walker or start from standing position. Make sure you note this for progression. | **Normal Range seconds**<br><table><tr><th>Age</th><th>Men</th><th>Women</th></tr><tr><td>60-64</td><td>5.6-3.8</td><td>6.0-4.4</td></tr><tr><td>65-69</td><td>5.9-4.3</td><td>6.4-4.8</td></tr><tr><td>70-74</td><td>6.2-4.4</td><td>7.1-4.9</td></tr><tr><td>75-79</td><td>7.2-4.6</td><td>7.4-5.2</td></tr><tr><td>80-84</td><td>7.6-5.2</td><td>8.7-5.7</td></tr><tr><td>85-89</td><td>8.9-5.5</td><td>9.6-6.2</td></tr><tr><td>90-94</td><td>10.0-6.2</td><td>11.5-7.3</td></tr></table> |

| TEST AND PURPOSE | PICTURE | EQUIPMENT NEEDED | EXPLANATION | RESULTS |
|---|---|---|---|---|
| **Narrow Stance**<br><br>Balance progression | | Wall, counter or chair within arm's reach for support if needed<br>Stopwatch or clock within view with second hand | Keep your feet together and stand for up to one minute.<br><br>*Time stops if loss of balance with need to hold on to support. | One minute: Normal *Progress to Staggered Stance Test*<br>*Less than 30 seconds: Continue balance program with wider stance and progress to narrow stance using support. (See Balance) |
| **Staggered Stance**<br><br>Balance progression | | Wall, counter or chair within arm's reach for support if needed<br>Stopwatch or clock within view with second hand | Stand with one foot in front of the other and slightly off to the side. Stand for up to one minute.<br>Repeat on other side for comparison<br>*Time stops if loss of balance with need to hold on to support. | One minute: Normal *Progress to Tandem Stance Test*<br>*Less than 30 seconds: Continue balance program using support. (See Balance) |
| **Tandem Stance**<br><br>Balance progression | | Wall, counter or chair within arm's reach for support if needed<br><br>Stopwatch or clock within view with second hand | Stand with one foot directly in back of the other – toe should be touching the opposite heel. Hold for up to one minute.<br><br>Repeat on other side for comparison<br><br>*Time stops if loss of balance with need to hold on to support. | One minute: Normal *Progress to One Leg Standing Balance*<br>*Less than 30 seconds: Continue balance program using support. (See Balance) |
| **Single Leg Stance**<br><br>Balance progression | | Wall, counter or chair within arm's reach for support if needed<br><br>Stopwatch or clock within view with second hand | Stand on one leg for up to one minute.<br><br>Repeat on other side for comparison<br><br>*Time stops if loss of balance with need to hold on to support or if opposite foot taps the floor | One minute: Normal<br><br>*Less than 30 seconds: Continue balance program using support. (See Balance) |

| EXERCISE<br><br>Myofascial Release | EXERCISE NUMBER | PAGE | REPS | SETS | X DAY | HOLD |
|---|---|---|---|---|---|---|
| ANTERIOR CHEST - BALL | 1 | | | | | |
| ANTERIOR CHEST - FOAM ROLL | 2 | | | | | |
| LATISSIMUS DORSI – BALL | 3 | | | | | |
| LATISSIMUS DORSI - FOAM ROLL | 4 | | | | | |
| TRICEP – FOAM ROLL | 5 | | | | | |
| OCCIPITAL RELEASE - FOAM ROLL | 6 | | | | | |
| THORACIC MOBILIZATION – SUPINE - FOAM ROLL | 7 | | | | | |
| THORACIC MOBILIZATION – STANDING - FOAM ROLL | 8 | | | | | |
| LUMBAR – STANDING – BALL - can do with foam roll | 9 | | | | | |
| LUMBAR – SUPINE – FOAM ROLLER | 10 | | | | | |
| HIP FLEXORS - BALL | 11 | | | | | |
| HIP FLEXORS – FOAM ROLL | 12 | | | | | |
| QUADRICEPS – BILATERAL - FOAM ROLL | 13 | | | | | |
| QUADRICEP – SINGLE - FOAM ROLL | 14 | | | | | |
| GLUTE /PIRIFORMIS - FOAM ROLL | 15 | | | | | |
| HIP ADDUCTORS – FOAM ROLL | 16 | | | | | |
| HAMSTRING – BILATERAL - FOAM ROLL | 17 | | | | | |
| HAMSTRING – SINGLE – FOAM ROLL | 18 | | | | | |
| CALVES – BILATERAL - FOAM ROLL | 19 | | | | | |
| CALVES – SINGLE - FOAM ROLL | 20 | | | | | |
| ILIOTIBIAL BAND (IT Band) - FOAM ROLL | 21 | | | | | |
| ILIOTIBIAL BAND (IT Band) - BALL | 22 | | | | | |
| PLANTAR FASCIA ROLLING – BALL | 23 | | | | | |
| PLANTAR FASCIA ROLLING - COLD SODA CAN | 24 | | | | | |

| EXERCISE<br><br>**Flexibility (Stretching)** | EXERCISE NUMBER | PAGE | REPS | SETS | X DAY | HOLD |
|---|---|---|---|---|---|---|
| INVERSION | 1 | | | | | |
| EVERSION | 2 | | | | | |
| ANTERIOR TIBIALIS | 3 | | | | | |
| PLANTARFLEXION | 4 | | | | | |
| DORSIFLEXION - STRAP | 5 | | | | | |
| DORSIFLEXION - FLOOR ASSISTED | 6 | | | | | |
| STANDING CALF STRETCH - GASTROC | 7 | | | | | |
| STANDING CALF STRETCH - GASTROC – HAND ON KNEE | 8 | | | | | |
| GASTROCNEMIUS STAIR STRETCH | 9 | | | | | |
| STANDING CALF STRETCH - SOLEUS | 10 | | | | | |
| HAMSTRING STRETCH – TOWEL, BAND, STRAP or BELT | 11 | | | | | |
| HAMSTRING STRETCH – TOWEL, BAND, STRAP or BELT | 12 | | | | | |
| HAMSTRING STRETCH - TABLE, BED OR COUCH | 13 | | | | | |
| HAMSTRING / KNEE EXTENSION STRETCH - SEATED | 14 | | | | | |
| HAMSTRING STRETCH - STANDING | 15 | | | | | |
| TOE TOUCH – STANDING - NARROW or WIDE BOS | 16 | | | | | |
| HEEL SLIDES - SELF ASSISTED | 17 | | | | | |
| HEEL SLIDES - LONG SIT ASSISTED - TOWEL, BAND, STRAP or BELT | 18 | | | | | |
| HEEL SLIDES - SUPINE | 19 | | | | | |
| KNEE BENDS - EXERCISE BALL | 20 | | | | | |
| KNEE FLEXION – SELF ASSISTED - PRONE | 21 | | | | | |
| KNEE FLEXION – BELT ASSISTED - PRONE | 22 | | | | | |
| HEEL SLIDES - SELF ASSISTED | 23 | | | | | |
| HEEL SLIDES - SEATED | 24 | | | | | |
| KNEE FLEXION – SCOOT FORWARD - SEATED | 25 | | | | | |

| EXERCISE<br><br>Flexibility (Stretching) | EXERCISE NUMBER | PAGE | REPS | SETS | X DAY | HOLD |
|---|---|---|---|---|---|---|
| KNEE FLEXION – STAIR OR STEP | 26 | | | | | |
| PIRIFORMIS STRETCH | 27 | | | | | |
| PIRIFORMIS STRETCH - EXERCISE BALL | 28 | | | | | |
| PIRIFORMIS STRETCH - LONG SIT | 29 | | | | | |
| PIRIFORMIS STRETCH – STANDING | 30 | | | | | |
| HIP FLEXOR STRETCH - SIDE OF BALL or CHAIR | 31 | | | | | |
| HIP FLEXOR STRETCH - STANDING | 32 | | | | | |
| HIP FLEXOR STRETCH - HALF KNEEL | 33 | | | | | |
| RUNNER'S STRETCH - MODIFIED | 34 | | | | | |
| HIP FLEXOR STRETCH – SUPINE | 35 | | | | | |
| HIP FLEXOR STRETCH – SUPINE - 2 | 36 | | | | | |
| QUAD STRETCH - SIDELYING | 37 | | | | | |
| QUAD STRETCH - STANDING | 38 | | | | | |
| KNEE FALL OUT STRETCH or FROG STRETCH | 39 | | | | | |
| BUTTERFLY STRETCH | 40 | | | | | |
| HIP ADDUCTOR STRECH – KNEELING | 41 | | | | | |
| HIP ADDUCTOR STRECH - STANDING | 42 | | | | | |
| HIP EXTERNAL ROTATION STRETCH - SUPINE | 43 | | | | | |
| HIP INTERNAL ROTATION STRETCH - SEATED | 44 | | | | | |
| IT BAND STRETCH - STANDING | 45 | | | | | |
| IT BAND STRETCH -- SIDELYING | 46 | | | | | |
| NECK ROTATION and SIDE BENDS | 47 | | | | | |
| NECK FLEXION AND EXTENSION | 48 | | | | | |
| TRUNK FLEXION - SEATED | 49 | | | | | |
| LOW BACK STRETCH - SEATED | 50 | | | | | |
| LOW BACK STRETCH – STANDING - STRAIGHT & LATERAL | 51 | | | | | |
| LOW BACK STRETCH – RAIL OR DOORKNOB | 52 | | | | | |

| EXERCISE<br><br>**Flexibility (Stretching)** | EXERCISE NUMBER | PAGE | REPS | SETS | X DAY | HOLD |
|---|---|---|---|---|---|---|
| PRAYER STRETCH and LATERAL | 53 | | | | | |
| PRAYER STRETCH - EXERCISE BALL | 54 | | | | | |
| CAT AND CAMEL | 55 | | | | | |
| KNEE TO CHEST STRETCH - SINGLE and BILATERAL | 56 | | | | | |
| PRONE ON ELBOWS | 57 | | | | | |
| PRESS UPS | 58 | | | | | |
| TRUNK ROTATION STRETCH – SINGLE LEG | 59 | | | | | |
| LOWER TRUNK ROTATIONS – BILATERAL | 60 | | | | | |
| TRUNK ROTATION - SEATED | 61 | | | | | |
| TRUNK ROTATION - STANDING or SEATED – DOWEL | 62 | | | | | |
| LATERAL TRUNK STRETCH - SINGLE, SEATED or STANDING | 63 | | | | | |
| LATERAL TRUNK STRETCH - BILATERAL SEATED or STANDING | 64 | | | | | |
| FLEXION  - SUPINE - DOWEL | 65 | | | | | |
| WALL WALK | 66 | | | | | |
| FLEXION - TABLE SLIDE | 67 | | | | | |
| FLEXION - TABLE SLIDE -  BALL | 68 | | | | | |
| EXTERNAL ROTATION - SUPINE – DOWEL<br>*INTERNAL ROTATION ON OPPOSITE ARM* | 69 | | | | | |
| EXTERNAL ROTATION - 90-90 - DOWEL | 70 | | | | | |
| EXTERNAL ROTATION – SEATED – DOWEL<br>*INTERNAL ROTATION ON OPPOSITE ARM* | 71 | | | | | |
| EXTERNAL ROTATION – STANDING – DOWEL<br>*INTERNAL ROTATION ON OPPOSITE ARM* | 72 | | | | | |
| ABDUCTION - TABLE SLIDE - BALL | 75 | | | | | |
| ABDUCTION WITH DOWEL | 76 | | | | | |
| LYING DOWN EXTENSION - TABLE or BED | 77 | | | | | |
| WAND EXTENSION - STANDING | 78 | | | | | |
| CHEST STRETCH – SEATED,  STANDING, or SUPINE | 79 | | | | | |

**Worksheets**

| EXERCISE<br><br>Flexibility (Stretching) | EXERCISE NUMBER | PAGE | REPS | SETS | X DAY | HOLD |
|---|---|---|---|---|---|---|
| TRICEP STRETCH - STRAP or TOWEL | 82 | | | | | |
| POSTERIOR SHOULDER/DELTOID RELEASE | 83 | | | | | |
| POSTERIOR CAPSULE STRETCH | 84 | | | | | |

| EXERCISE<br>Core / Stability | EXERCISE NUMBER | PAGE | REPS | SETS | X DAY | HOLD |
|---|---|---|---|---|---|---|
| ABDOMINAL BRACING TRAINING | 1 | | | | | |
| ABDOMINAL BRACING - SUPINE | 2 | | | | | |
| PELVIC TILT - SUPINE | 3 | | | | | |
| PELVIC TILT - KNEELING | 4 | | | | | |
| BRIDGING | 5 | | | | | |
| BRIDGE - BOSU | 6 | | | | | |
| BRIDGING WITH PILLOW SQUEEZE | 7 | | | | | |
| BRIDGING WITH PILLOW SQUEEZE - BOSU | 8 | | | | | |
| BRACE SUPINE MARCHING / BRIDGE LEG UP | 9 | | | | | |
| BRIDGE LEG UP - BOSU - | 10 | | | | | |
| SINGLE LEG BRIDGE | 11 | | | | | |
| BRIDGE SINGLE LEG - BOSU | 12 | | | | | |
| BRIDGING CROSSED LEG | 13 | | | | | |
| BRIDGING CROSSED LEG – BOSU | 14 | | | | | |
| BRIDGING CROSSED LEG - ARMS UP | 15 | | | | | |
| BRIDGING CROSSED LEG - ARMS UP - BOSU | 16 | | | | | |
| BRIDGE - ELASTIC BAND | 17 | | | | | |
| BRIDGING - ABDUCTION - ELASTIC BAND | 18 | | | | | |
| FLOOR BRIDGE - EXERCISE BALL | 19 | | | | | |
| FLOOR BRIDGE ALTERNATE LEG LIFT - EXERCISE BALL | 20 | | | | | |
| BRIDGE UPPER BACK - EXERCISE BALL | 21 | | | | | |
| BRIDGE UPPER BACK - SINGLE LEG - EXERCISE BALL | 22 | | | | | |
| QUADRUPED ALTERNATE ARM | 23 | | | | | |
| QUADRUPED ALTERNATE LEG | 24 | | | | | |
| QUADRUPED ALTERNATE ARM AND LEG | 25 | | | | | |
| BIRD DOG ELBOW TOUCHES | 26 | | | | | |

| EXERCISE Core / Stability | EXERCISE NUMBER | PAGE | REPS | SETS | X DAY | HOLD |
|---|---|---|---|---|---|---|
| PRONE BALL | 27 | | | | | |
| PRONE BALL - ALTERNATE ARM | 28 | | | | | |
| PRONE BALL - ALTERNATE LEG | 29 | | | | | |
| PRONE BALL - ALTERNATE ARM AND LEG | 30 | | | | | |
| MODIFIED PLANK | 31 | | | | | |
| MODIFIED PLANK - ALTERNATE LEG | 32 | | | | | |
| FULL PLANK | 33 | | | | | |
| PLANK - ALTERNATE ARMS | 34 | | | | | |
| PLANK - ALTERNATE LEGS | 35 | | | | | |
| PLANK - EXERCISE BALL | 36 | | | | | |
| PRONE ON ELBOWS | 37 | | | | | |
| PRESS UPS | 38 | | | | | |
| SKYDIVER | 39 | | | | | |
| PRONE SUPERMAN - BOSU | 40 | | | | | |
| TRUNK EXTENSION - BOSU | 41 | | | | | |
| TRUNK EXTENSION - HANDS CROSSED IN FRONT - BOSU | 43 | | | | | |
| SUPERMAN - ARMS BACK- EXERCISE BALL | 44 | | | | | |
| SUPERMAN – BOTH ARMS IN FRONT - EXERCISE BALL | 45 | | | | | |
| SUPERMAN – ONE ARM FORWARD / ONE ARM BACK - EXERCISE BALL | 46 | | | | | |
| LATERAL PLANK MODIFIED | 47 | | | | | |
| LATERAL PLANK MODIFIED- BOSU | 48 | | | | | |
| LATERAL PLANK - 1 KNEE 1 FOOT | 49 | | | | | |
| LATERAL PLANK - 1 KNEE 1 FOOT – BOSU | 50 | | | | | |
| LATERAL PLANK | 51 | | | | | |
| LATERAL PLANK - BOSU | 52 | | | | | |

| EXERCISE | EXERCISE NUMBER | PAGE | REPS | SETS | X DAY | HOLD |
|---|---|---|---|---|---|---|
| Core / Stability | | | | | | |
| LEAN BACK | 53 | | | | | |
| LEAN BACK - BOSU | 54 | | | | | |
| LEAN BACK WITH ARMS OUT | 55 | | | | | |
| LEAN BACK WITH ARMS OUT - BOSU | 56 | | | | | |
| LEAN BACK WITH TWIST | 57 | | | | | |
| LEAN BACK WITH TWIST – BOSU | 58 | | | | | |
| CRUNCHY FROG | 59 | | | | | |
| SEATED BIKE - FORWARD AND BACKWARDS | 60 | | | | | |
| CRUNCH – ARMS OUT | 61 | | | | | |
| CRUNCH – ARMS OUT - BOSU | 62 | | | | | |
| CRUNCH – ARMS IN BACK OF HEAD | 63 | | | | | |
| CRUNCH – ARMS IN BACK OF HEAD - BOSU | 64 | | | | | |
| OBLIQUE CRUNCH | 65 | | | | | |
| OBLIQUE CRUNCH - BOSU | 66 | | | | | |
| 90 DEGREE CRUNCH | 67 | | | | | |
| BALL CRUNCH – Can put legs on seat of chair | 68 | | | | | |
| CURL UPS – ARMS ON LEGS - EXERCISE BALL | 69 | | | | | |
| CURL UPS- ARMS CROSSED IN FRONT - EXERCISE BALL | 70 | | | | | |
| CURL UPS – ARMS BEHIND HEAD - EXERCISE BALL | 71 | | | | | |
| SUPINE CRUNCH TOUCH - EXERCISE BALL | 72 | | | | | |
| LOWER ABDOMINAL CRUNCH – WITH or WITHOUT BALL | 73 | | | | | |
| HIGH MARCH CRUNCH | 74 | | | | | |
| STANDING SIDE CRUNCH | 75 | | | | | |
| STANDING BIKE CRUNCH | 76 | | | | | |

| EXERCISE<br><br>Lower Extremity - Lying & Seated Strengthening and Range of Motion | EXERCISE NUMBER | PAGE | REPS | SETS | X DAY | HOLD |
|---|---|---|---|---|---|---|
| INVERSION – SEATED - ELASTIC BAND | 1 | | | | | |
| INVERSION – SEATED - ELASTIC BAND - 2 | 2 | | | | | |
| EVERSION – SEATED - ELASTIC BAND | 3 | | | | | |
| EVERSION – SEATED - ELASTIC BAND - 2 | 4 | | | | | |
| ANKLE PUMPS - SEATED | 5 | | | | | |
| ANKLE PUMPS – SUPINE or FEET UP ON STOOL | 6 | | | | | |
| DORSIFLEXION – SEATED - ELASTIC BAND | 7 | | | | | |
| DORSIFLEXION – SEATED - ELASTIC BAND - 2 | 8 | | | | | |
| PLANTARFLEXION - STRAP | 9 | | | | | |
| PLANTARFLEXION - SEATED – ELASTIC BAND | 10 | | | | | |
| HEEL SLIDES - SUPINE | 11 | | | | | |
| HEEL SLIDES - RESISTED EXTENSION – ELASTIC BAND | 12 | | | | | |
| QUAD SET –ISOMETRIC | 13 | | | | | |
| QUAD SET WITH TOWEL UNDER HEEL - ISOMETRIC | 14 | | | | | |
| SHORT ARC QUAD (SAQ) – SELF ASSISTED | 15 | | | | | |
| SHORT ARC QUAD - (SAQ) | 16 | | | | | |
| KNEE EXTENSION - SELF ASSISTED | 17 | | | | | |
| PARTIAL ARC QUAD - LOW SEAT | 18 | | | | | |
| LONG ARC QUAD (LAQ) – LOW SEAT (90 deg) | 19 | | | | | |
| LONG ARC QUAD (LAQ) – LOW SEAT - ANKLE WEIGHTS | 20 | | | | | |
| LONG ARC QUAD (LAQ) - HIGH SEAT | 21 | | | | | |
| LONG ARC QUAD (LAQ) - HIGH SEAT - ANKLE WEIGHTS | 22 | | | | | |
| LONG ARC QUAD - ELASTIC BAND – HAND HELD | 23 | | | | | |
| LONG ARC QUAD - ELASTIC BAND | 24 | | | | | |

| EXERCISE<br><br>Lower Extremity - Lying & Seated Strengthening and Range of Motion | EXERCISE NUMBER | PAGE | REPS | SETS | X DAY | HOLD |
|---|---|---|---|---|---|---|
| HAMSTRING CURLS - PRONE - ASSISTED | 25 | | | | | |
| HAMSTRING CURLS - PRONE | 26 | | | | | |
| HAMSTRING CURLS - - PRONE - WEIGHTS | 27 | | | | | |
| HAMSTRING CURLS – PRONE - ELASTIC BAND | 28 | | | | | |
| HAMSTRING CURLS – ELASTIC BAND | 29 | | | | | |
| HAMSTRING CURLS – ELASTIC BAND - 2 | 30 | | | | | |
| HAMSTRING CURLS ON BALL | 31 | | | | | |
| HAMSTRING CURLS - SINGLE LEG - EXERCISE BALL | 32 | | | | | |
| HIP FLEXION ISOMETRIC | 33 | | | | | |
| HIP FLEXION ISOMETRIC BILATERAL | 34 | | | | | |
| HIP FLEXION – ISOMETRIC | 35 | | | | | |
| STRAIGHT LEG RAISE (SLR) | 36 | | | | | |
| STRAIGHT LEG RAISE (SLR) – ANKLE WEIGHTS | 37 | | | | | |
| STRAIGHT LEG RAISE (SLR) - ELASTIC BAND | 38 | | | | | |
| SEATED MARCHING | 39 | | | | | |
| SEATED MARCHING - ELASTIC BAND | 40 | | | | | |
| HIP EXTENSION - PRONE | 41 | | | | | |
| HIP EXTENSION – PRONE – ANKLE WEIGHTS | 42 | | | | | |
| HIP EXTENSION – PRONE – ELASTIC BAND | 43 | | | | | |
| HIP EXTENSION – QUADRUPED | 44 | | | | | |
| HIP ABDUCTION - SUPINE | 45 | | | | | |
| HIP ABDUCTION - SUPINE – ANKLE WEIGHTS | 46 | | | | | |
| HIP ABDUCTION – SUPINE - ELASTIC BAND | 47 | | | | | |
| HIP ABDUCTION / CLAMS– SUPINE - ELASTIC BAND | 48 | | | | | |
| MODIFIED HIP ABDUCTION – SIDELYING | 49 | | | | | |

**Worksheets**

| EXERCISE<br><br>Lower Extremity - Lying & Seated Strengthening and Range of Motion | EXERCISE NUMBER | PAGE | REPS | SETS | X DAY | HOLD |
|---|---|---|---|---|---|---|
| HIP ABDUCTION – SIDELYING | 50 | | | | | |
| HIP ABDUCTION – SIDELYING - WEIGHTS | 51 | | | | | |
| HIP ABDUCTION – SIDELYING - ELASTIC BAND | 52 | | | | | |
| CLAM SHELLS | 53 | | | | | |
| SIDELYING CLAM - ELASTIC BAND | 54 | | | | | |
| HIP ABDUCTION - FIRE HYDRANT - QUADRUPED | 55 | | | | | |
| HIP ABDUCTION - FIRE HYDRANT – QUADRUPED - ELASTIC BAND | 56 | | | | | |
| HIP ABDUCTION - SEATED - STRAIGHT LEG | 57 | | | | | |
| HIP ABDUCTION - SEATED - STRAIGHT LEG – ANKLE WEIGHT | 58 | | | | | |
| HIP ABDUCTION - SINGLE- SEATED | 59 | | | | | |
| HIP ABDUCTION - SINGLE- SEATED – ELASTIC BAND | 60 | | | | | |
| HIP ABDUCTION - BILATERAL- SEATED | 61 | | | | | |
| HIP ABDUCTION - BILATERAL- SEATED - ELASTIC BAND | 62 | | | | | |
| HIP ADDUCTION SQUEEZE – SUPINE – KNEES BENT | 63 | | | | | |
| HIP ADDUCTION SQUEEZE – SUPINE – LEGS STRAIGHT | 64 | | | | | |
| HIP ADDUCTION - SIDELYING | 65 | | | | | |
| INTERNAL ROTATION - HEEL SQUEEZE - ISOMETRIC | 67 | | | | | |
| HIP INTERNAL ROTATION - SUPINE | 68 | | | | | |
| REVERSE CLAMS - SIDELYING | 69 | | | | | |
| REVERSE CLAMS - SIDELYING  - ELASTIC BAND | 70 | | | | | |
| HIP INTERNAL ROTATION  - SEATED | 71 | | | | | |
| HIP INTERNAL ROTATION - ELASTIC BAND | 72 | | | | | |
| HIP EXTERNAL ROTATION - SUPINE | 73 | | | | | |

**Worksheets**

| EXERCISE<br><br>Lower Extremity - Lying & Seated Strengthening and Range of Motion | EXERCISE NUMBER | PAGE | REPS | SETS | X DAY | HOLD |
|---|---|---|---|---|---|---|
| HIP EXTERNAL ROTATION - ELASTIC BAND | 74 | | | | | |
| HIP ROTATIONS – BILATERAL - SIDELYING | 75 | | | | | |
| HIP ROTATION - SEATED - BALL and ELASTIC BAND | 76 | | | | | |
| PRESS – BILATERAL – ELASTIC BAND | 77 | | | | | |
| PRESS – SINGLE LEG – ELASTIC BAND | 78 | | | | | |
| HIP HIKE - STANDING | 79 | | | | | |
| HIP HIKE – KNEELING | 80 | | | | | |
| GLUTE SETS - PRONE | 81 | | | | | |
| GLUTE SET - SUPINE | 82 | | | | | |
| GLUTE SQUEEZE - SITTING | 83 | | | | | |
| GLUTE SCULPT (MAX/MEDIUS) | 84 | | | | | |

| EXERCISE<br><br>Upper Extremity<br>Strengthening and Range of Motion | EXERCISE NUMBER | PAGE | REPS | SETS | X DAY | HOLD |
|---|---|---|---|---|---|---|
| ELBOW FLEXION EXTENSION - SUPINE | 1 | | | | | |
| ELBOW FLEXION / EXTENSION - GRAVITY ELIMINATED | 2 | | | | | |
| BICEPS CURLS – ALTERNATING | 3 | | | | | |
| BICEPS CURL - SELF FIXATION – ELASTIC BAND | 4 | | | | | |
| SEATED BICEPS CURLS - ALTERNATING | 5 | | | | | |
| SEATED BICEPS CURLS - BILATERAL | 6 | | | | | |
| CONCENTRATION CURLS – SITTING | 7 | | | | | |
| PREACHER CURL ON BALL | 8 | | | | | |
| BICEPS CURLS | 9 | | | | | |
| BICEPS CURLS - RADIOBRACHIALIS - HAMMER CURL | 10 | | | | | |
| BICEPS CURLS - BRACHIALIS | 11 | | | | | |
| BICEPS CURLS – ROTATE OUTWARD | 12 | | | | | |
| BICEPS CURLS – ONE ARM - ELASTIC BAND | 13 | | | | | |
| BICEPS CURLS – BILATERAL - ELASTIC BAND | 14 | | | | | |
| BICEPS CURLS - RADIOBRACHIALIS - HAMMER CURL – ONE ARM - ELASTIC BAND | 15 | | | | | |
| BICEPS CURLS - RADIOBRACHIALIS - HAMMER CURL – BILATERAL - ELASTIC BAND | 16 | | | | | |
| BICEPS CURLS – BRACHIALIS - ONE ARM - ELASTIC BAND | 17 | | | | | |
| BICEPS CURL – BRACHIALIS – BILATERAL - ELASTIC BAND | 18 | | | | | |
| TRICEPS - SELF FIXATION - ELASTIC BAND | 19 | | | | | |
| OVERHEAD TRICEPS - SELF FIXATION –SEATED OR STANDING - ELASTIC BAND | 20 | | | | | |
| TRICEP EXTENSION – SITTING OR STANDING - WEIGHT | 21 | | | | | |
| TRICEP EXTENSION – SITTING OR STANDING – BILATERAL - WEIGHT | 22 | | | | | |
| ELBOW EXTENSION - BALL | 23 | | | | | |

| EXERCISE<br><br>Upper Extremity<br>Strengthening and Range of Motion | EXERCISE NUMBER | PAGE | REPS | SETS | X DAY | HOLD |
|---|---|---|---|---|---|---|
| ELBOW EXTENSION - SKULL CRUSHER - BALL | 24 | | | | | |
| TRICEPS - ELASTIC BAND | 25 | | | | | |
| TRICEPS - BENT OVER | 26 | | | | | |
| CHAIR DIPS / PUSH UPS | 27 | | | | | |
| DIPS OFF CHAIR | 28 | | | | | |
| PENDULUM SHOULDER FORWARD/BACK | 29 | | | | | |
| PENDULUM SHOULDER – SIDE TO SIDE | 30 | | | | | |
| PENDULUM SHOULDER CIRCLES | 31 | | | | | |
| PENDULUMS - SUPINE | 32 | | | | | |
| ISOMETRIC FLEXION | 33 | | | | | |
| SHOULDER FLEXION – SIDELYING | 34 | | | | | |
| FLEXION – SUPINE  - SINGLE OR BILATERAL | 35 | | | | | |
| FLEXION – SUPINE – SINGLE OR BILATERAL - WEIGHT | 36 | | | | | |
| FLEXION – SUPINE -  DOWEL | 37 | | | | | |
| FLEXION – SUPINE - DOWEL - Weight | 38 | | | | | |
| FLEXION - SELF FIXATION – ELASTIC BAND | 39 | | | | | |
| FLEXION – ELASTIC BAND | 40 | | | | | |
| FLEXION - STANDING - PALMS DOWN / OVERHAND DOWEL | 41 | | | | | |
| FLEXION - STANDING - PALMS UP / UNDERHAND DOWEL | 42 | | | | | |
| FLEXION – PALMS FACING INWARD | 43 | | | | | |
| FLEXION – PALMS DOWN | 44 | | | | | |
| V RAISE | 45 | | | | | |
| V RAISE – WEIGHTS | 46 | | | | | |
| MILITARY PRESS – DOWEL | 47 | | | | | |
| MILITARY PRESS - FREE WEIGHTS | 48 | | | | | |

**Worksheets**

| EXERCISE<br>**Upper Extremity<br>Strengthening and Range of Motion** | EXERCISE NUMBER | PAGE | REPS | SETS | X DAY | HOLD |
|---|---|---|---|---|---|---|
| ISOMETRIC EXTENSION | 49 | | | | | |
| PRONE EXTENSION - EXERCISE BALL | 50 | | | | | |
| SHOULDER EXTENSION - STANDING | 51 | | | | | |
| SHOULDER EXTENSION - STANDING - WEIGHTS | 52 | | | | | |
| EXTENSION – STANDING – DOWEL | 53 | | | | | |
| EXTENSION - SELF FIXATION - ELASTIC BAND | 54 | | | | | |
| EXTENSION - ELASTIC BAND | 55 | | | | | |
| EXTENSION - BILATERAL - ELASTIC BAND | 56 | | | | | |
| INTERNAL ROTATION – ISOMETRIC | 57 | | | | | |
| INTERNAL ROTATION - ISOMETRIC- ELEVATED | 58 | | | | | |
| INTERNAL ROTATION - SIDELYING | 59 | | | | | |
| INTERNAL ROTATION - ELASTIC BAND | 60 | | | | | |
| INTERNAL / EXTERNAL ROTATION - STANDING – DOWEL | 61 | | | | | |
| INTERNAL ROTATION – DOWEL | 62 | | | | | |
| EXTERNAL ROTATION - ISOMETRIC | 63 | | | | | |
| EXTERNAL ROTATION - ISOMETRIC – ELEVATED | 64 | | | | | |
| EXTERNAL ROTATION WITH TOWEL - SIDELYING | 65 | | | | | |
| EXTERNAL ROTATION – 90/90 - WEIGHTS | 66 | | | | | |
| EXTERNAL ROTATION - BILATERAL - ELASTIC BAND | 67 | | | | | |
| EXTERNAL ROTATION - ELASTIC BAND | 68 | | | | | |
| ADDUCTION – ISOMETRIC | 69 | | | | | |
| ADDUCTION - ELASTIC BAND | 70 | | | | | |
| ABDUCTION – ISOMETRIC | 71 | | | | | |
| HORIZONTAL ABDUCTION - DOWEL | 72 | | | | | |

| EXERCISE<br><br>**Upper Extremity**<br>**Strengthening and Range of Motion** | EXERCISE NUMBER | PAGE | REPS | SETS | X DAY | HOLD |
|---|---|---|---|---|---|---|
| HORIZONTAL ABDUCTION/ADDUCTTION - SUPINE | 73 | | | | | |
| HORIZONTAL ABDUCTION/ADDUCTTION - SUPINE -WEIGHT | 74 | | | | | |
| ABDUCTION - SIDELYING | 75 | | | | | |
| HORIZONTAL ABDUCTION - SIDELYING | 76 | | | | | |
| ABDUCTION – WEIGHT | 77 | | | | | |
| ABDUCTION – ELASTIC BAND | 78 | | | | | |
| HORIZONTAL ABDUCTION – BILATERAL - ELASTIC BAND | 79 | | | | | |
| 90/90 ABDUCTION - WEIGHT | 80 | | | | | |
| LATERAL RAISES | 81 | | | | | |
| LATERAL RAISES – LEAN FORWARD | 82 | | | | | |
| LATERAL RAISES – LEAN FORWARD - ARM ROTATION | 83 | | | | | |
| FRONTAL RAISE – WEIGHTS | 84 | | | | | |
| UPRIGHT ROW – WEIGHTS | 85 | | | | | |
| UPRIGHT ROW – ELASTIC BAND | 86 | | | | | |
| SHRUGS | 87 | | | | | |
| SHRUGS - WEIGHTS | 88 | | | | | |
| SHOULDER ROLLS | 89 | | | | | |
| SHOULDER ROLLS - WEIGHTS | 90 | | | | | |
| SCAPULAR RETRACTIONS - BILATERAL | 91 | | | | | |
| SCAPULAR RETRACTION – SINGLE ARM | 92 | | | | | |
| ELASTIC BAND SCAPULAR RETRACTIONS WITH MINI SHOULDER EXTENSIONS | 93 | | | | | |
| PRONE RETRACTION | 94 | | | | | |
| SCAPULAR PROTRACTION - SUPINE - BILATERAL | 95 | | | | | |
| SCAPULAR PROTRACTION - SUPINE - WEIGHT | 96 | | | | | |

| EXERCISE<br><br>Upper Extremity<br>Strengthening and Range of Motion | EXERCISE NUMBER | PAGE | REPS | SETS | X DAY | HOLD |
|---|---|---|---|---|---|---|
| SCAPULAR PROTRACTION - SUPINE - ELASTIC BAND | 97 | | | | | |
| SCAPULAR PROTRACTION / TABLE PLANK | 98 | | | | | |
| CHEST PRESS – SEATED or STANDING - ELASTIC BAND | 99 | | | | | |
| CHEST PRESS – BALL, FLOOR or BENCH-WEIGHTS | 100 | | | | | |
| DOWEL PRESS – STANDING | 101 | | | | | |
| CHEST PRESS – STANDING or SEATED | 102 | | | | | |
| BENT OVER ROWS | 103 | | | | | |
| ROWS – PRONE | 104 | | | | | |
| ROWS - ELASTIC BAND | 105 | | | | | |
| WIDE ROWS - ELASTIC BAND | 106 | | | | | |
| LOW ROW – ELASTIC BAND | 107 | | | | | |
| HIGH ROW – ELASTIC BAND | 108 | | | | | |
| FLY'S – FLOOR - WEIGHT | 109 | | | | | |
| FLY'S – BALL or BENCH – WEIGHT | 110 | | | | | |
| WALL PUSH UPS | 111 | | | | | |
| WALL PUSH UP - BALL | 112 | | | | | |
| WALL PUSH UP - Triceps uneven | 113 | | | | | |
| WALL PUSH UP - Hands inverted | 114 | | | | | |
| WALL PUSH UP - Narrow | 115 | | | | | |
| WALL PUSH UP – Wide | 116 | | | | | |
| PUSH UPS - BALL | 117 | | | | | |
| PUSH UP - MODIFIED | 118 | | | | | |
| PUSH UP | 119 | | | | | |
| PUSH UP -DIAMOND | 120 | | | | | |
| PUSH UP – MODIFIED - BOSU - UNSTABLE | 121 | | | | | |

**Worksheets**

| EXERCISE<br><br>Upper Extremity<br>Strengthening and Range of Motion | EXERCISE NUMBER | PAGE | REPS | SETS | X DAY | HOLD |
|---|---|---|---|---|---|---|
| PUSH UP – BOSU - UNSTABLE | 122 | | | | | |
| PUSH UP – MODIFIED – INVERTED BOSU - UNSTABLE | 123 | | | | | |
| PUSH UP – INVERTED BOSU - UNSTABLE | 124 | | | | | |

| EXERCISE<br><br>**Balance / Standing Exercises** | EXERCISE NUMBER | PAGE | REPS | SETS | X DAY | HOLD |
|---|---|---|---|---|---|---|
| WIDE BOS DECREASING TO NARROW BOS | 1 | | | | | |
| NARROW BOS | 2 | | | | | |
| ARM MOVEMENT | 3 | | | | | |
| TRUNK ROTATION | 4 | | | | | |
| EYES SHUTS | 5 | | | | | |
| HEAD TURNS | 6 | | | | | |
| READING ALOUD | 7 | | | | | |
| BALANCE PAD | 8 | | | | | |
| SPLIT STANCE – SEMI TANDEM | 9 | | | | | |
| SPLIT STANCE - *Progression* | 10 | | | | | |
| TANDEM- SHARPENED ROMBERG STANCE | 11 | | | | | |
| TANDEM STANCE - Progression | 12 | | | | | |
| SINGLE LEG STANCE (SLS) | 13 | | | | | |
| SINGLE LEG STANCE (SLS) - *Progression* | 14 | | | | | |
| SLS – LEG FORWARD | 15 | | | | | |
| SLS – LEG BACKWARDS | 16 | | | | | |
| SLS – LEG FORWARD / OPPOSITE ARM UP | 17 | | | | | |
| SLS – LEG BACKWARDS / OPPOSITE ARM UP | 18 | | | | | |
| SLS - REACH FORWARD | 19 | | | | | |
| SLS - REACH TWIST | 20 | | | | | |
| SINGLE LEG TOE TAP | 21 | | | | | |
| SINGLE LEG STANCE - CLOCKS | 22 | | | | | |
| BALL ROLLS - HEEL TOE | 23 | | | | | |
| BALL ROLLS - LATERAL | 24 | | | | | |
| SQUAT | 25 | | | | | |
| SIT TO STAND | 26 | | | | | |

| EXERCISE | EXERCISE NUMBER | PAGE | REPS | SETS | X DAY | HOLD |
|---|---|---|---|---|---|---|
| **Balance / Standing Exercises** | | | | | | |
| SQUATS – WALL WITH BALL | 27 | | | | | |
| SQUATS WITH WEIGHTS | 28 | | | | | |
| MINI SQUAT - UNSTABLE SUPPORT - FOAM PAD | 29 | | | | | |
| SQUATS - SINGLE LEG | 30 | | | | | |
| SIDE TO SIDE WEIGHT SHIFT | 31 | | | | | |
| FORWARD AND BACKWARDS WEIGHT SHIFTS | 32 | | | | | |
| SPLIT STANCE WEIGHT SHIFT SIDE TO SIDE | 33 | | | | | |
| SPLIT STANCE WEIGHT SHIFT FORWARD AND BACKWARDS | 34 | | | | | |
| WALL FALLS - FORWARD - BALANCE DRILL | 35 | | | | | |
| WALL FALLS - LATERAL - BALANCE DRILL | 36 | | | | | |
| WALL FALLS - BACKWARDS - BALANCE DRILL | 37 | | | | | |
| WALL FALLS - SINGLE LEG - FORWARD - BALANCE DRILL | 38 | | | | | |
| WALL FALLS - SINGLE LEG - LATERAL - BALANCE DRILL | 39 | | | | | |
| WALL FALLS - SINGLE LEG - MEDIAL - BALANCE DRILL | 40 | | | | | |
| WALL FALLS - SINGLE LEG - BACKWARDS - BALANCE DRILL | 41 | | | | | |
| FALL LATERAL - STEP RECOVERY | 42 | | | | | |
| FALL FORWARD - STEP RECOVERY | 43 | | | | | |
| FALL BACKWARD - STEP RECOVERY | 44 | | | | | |
| TOE TAP ABDUCTION | 45 | | | | | |
| HIP ABDUCTION - STANDING | 46 | | | | | |
| HIP EXTENSION – STANDING | 47 | | | | | |
| HIP FLEXION - STANDING – STRAIGHT LEG RAISE | 48 | | | | | |
| HIP / KNEE FLEXION - SINGLE LEG | 49 | | | | | |
| STANDING MARCHING | 50 | | | | | |

| EXERCISE<br><br>**Balance / Standing Exercises** | EXERCISE NUMBER | PAGE | REPS | SETS | X DAY | HOLD |
|---|---|---|---|---|---|---|
| HAMSTRING CURL | 51 | | | | | |
| TOE RAISES | 52 | | | | | |
| TOE RAISES IR AND ER | 53 | | | | | |
| ONE LEGGED TOE RAISE | 54 | | | | | |
| SINGLE LEG BALANCE FORWARD | 55 | | | | | |
| SINGLE LEG BALANCE LATERAL | 56 | | | | | |
| SINGLE LEG BALANCE RETRO | 57 | | | | | |
| SINGLE LEG STANCE RETROLATERAL | 58 | | | | | |
| SQUAT | 59 | | | | | |
| SINGLE LEG SQUAT | 60 | | | | | |
| LUNGE – STATIC | 61 | | | | | |
| LUNGE FORWARD/BACKWARD | 62 | | | | | |
| FOUR CORNER MARCHING IN PLACE | 63 | | | | | |
| FOUR CORNER MARCHING IN PLACE WITH HEAD TURNS | 64 | | | | | |
| WALKING ON HEELS FORWARD AND BACKWARDS | 65 | | | | | |
| WALKING ON TOES FORWARD AND BACKWARDS | 66 | | | | | |
| TANDEM STANCE AND WALK – FORWARD AND BACKWARDS | 67 | | | | | |
| RUNNING MAN | 68 | | | | | |
| HOP STICK - FORWARD | 69 | | | | | |
| HOP STICK - BACKWARDS | 70 | | | | | |
| MINI LATERAL LUNGE | 71 | | | | | |
| SIDE STEPPING | 72 | | | | | |
| HOP STICK - LATERAL | 73 | | | | | |
| SINGLE LEG DEAD LIFT | 74 | | | | | |

| EXERCISE<br><br>Balance / Standing Exercises | EXERCISE NUMBER | PAGE | REPS | SETS | X DAY | HOLD |
|---|---|---|---|---|---|---|
| CONE TAPS - SINGLE LEG STANCE | 75 | | | | | |
| CONE TAPS - SINGLE LEG STANCE - UNSTABLE | 76 | | | | | |
| FIGURE 8 AROUND CONES | 77 | | | | | |
| FIGURE 8 AROUND CONES – FOOT OR HAND TAP | 78 | | | | | |
| BALANCE DOUBLE LEG STANCE - WIDE | 79 | | | | | |
| BALANCE DOUBLE LEG STANCE - NARROW | 80 | | | | | |
| TANDEM STANCE | 81 | | | | | |
| TANDEM WALK | 82 | | | | | |
| SINGLE LEG STANCE - ABDUCTION | 83 | | | | | |
| SINGLE LEG STANCE - ABDUCTION | 84 | | | | | |
| SINGLE LEG STANCE – FORWARD KICK | 85 | | | | | |
| SINGLE LEG STANCE – HAMSTRING CURL | 86 | | | | | |
| SINGLE LEG SQUAT – LEG FORWARD | 87 | | | | | |
| SINGLE LEG SQUAT – LEG BACKWARDS | 88 | | | | | |
| TOE TAP OR HEEL PLACEMENT | 89 | | | | | |
| PULL UP FOOT TOUCHES ON STEP | 90 | | | | | |
| ALTERNATING SUSTAINED FOOT TOUCHES ON STEP | 91 | | | | | |
| STEP UP AND OVER | 92 | | | | | |
| FORWARD SWING THROUGH STEP | 93 | | | | | |
| SIDE STEPPING - *REPEAT STEPS 89-93 from a side approach.* | 94 | | | | | |

| EXERCISE<br><br>Agility/Reactivity/Speed | EXERCISE NUMBER | PAGE | REPS | SETS | X DAY | HOLD |
|---|---|---|---|---|---|---|
| Four Square Drills | 1 | | | | | |
| Dots | 2 | | | | | |
| Ladder Drills | 3 | | | | | |
| Box Drills | 4 | | | | | |
| Cones | 5 | | | | | |
| Hurdles | 6 | | | | | |

# Myofascial Release

Myofascial release (MFR, self-myofascial release) is an alternative medicine therapy that claims to treat skeletal muscle immobility and pain by relaxing contracted muscles, improving blood and lymphatic circulation, and stimulating the stretch reflex in muscles.

Fascia is a thin, tough, elastic type of connective tissue that wraps most structures within the human body, including muscle. Fascia supports and protects these structures. Osteopathic theory proposes that this soft tissue can become restricted due to psychogenic disease, overuse, trauma, infectious agents, or inactivity, often resulting in pain, muscle tension, and corresponding diminished blood flow. (Wikipedia - *https://en.wikipedia.org/wiki/Myofascial_release*)

## Possible Benefits of Myofascial Release

- Muscle relaxation
- Improves muscular and joint range of motion
- Reduces muscle soreness and improves tissue recovery
- Encourages the flow of lymph.
- Improves neuromuscular efficiency.
- Reduces adhesions and scar tissue.
- Releases trigger point (sensitivity and pain) – brings in blood flow and nutrient exchange.
- Maintains normal functional muscular length / Provides optimal length-tension relationship.
- Corrects muscle imbalances

## USE

- Roll on foam roller or ball until you find the sore spot or trigger point. When you find this point, stop and rest on it or decrease the range to this particular area and hold for 10-20 seconds.
- Apply pressure to muscle area only. Try not to roll over bones, joints or directly on the spine (you can use a ball over the muscles on the side of the spine).
- Use this as a part of your warmup for particular areas you are exercising that day (for instance the hamstrings, calves and quadricep on leg strengthening day)
- You can use this technique on additional days for trouble areas and can even devote a dedicated session for whole body myofascial release.

**Equipment Needed: FOAM ROLLER and/or TEXTURED or SOFT MASSAGE BALL**

| EXERCISE | EXERCISE NUMBER | NOTES |
|---|---|---|
| Myofascial Release | | |
| ANTERIOR CHEST - BALL | 1 | |
| ANTERIOR CHEST - FOAM ROLL | 2 | |
| LATISSIMUS DORSI – BALL | 3 | |
| LATISSIMUS DORSI - FOAM ROLL | 4 | |
| TRICEP – FOAM ROLL | 5 | |
| OCCIPITAL RELEASE - FOAM ROLL | 6 | |
| THORACIC MOBILIZATION – SUPINE - FOAM ROLL | 7 | |
| THORACIC MOBILIZATION – STANDING - FOAM ROLL | 8 | |
| LUMBAR – STANDING – BALL - can do with foam roll | 9 | |
| LUMBAR – SUPINE – FOAM ROLLER | 10 | |
| HIP FLEXORS - BALL | 11 | |
| HIP FLEXORS – FOAM ROLL | 12 | |
| QUADRICEPS – BILATERAL - FOAM ROLL | 13 | |
| QUADRICEP – SINGLE - FOAM ROLL | 14 | |
| GLUTE /PIRIFORMIS - FOAM ROLL | 15 | |
| HIP ADDUCTORS – FOAM ROLL | 16 | |
| HAMSTRING – BILATERAL - FOAM ROLL | 17 | |
| HAMSTRING – SINGLE – FOAM ROLL | 18 | |
| CALVES – BILATERAL - FOAM ROLL | 19 | |
| CALVES – SINGLE - FOAM ROLL | 20 | |
| ILIOTIBIAL BAND (IT Band) - FOAM ROLL | 21 | |
| ILIOTIBIAL BAND (IT Band) - BALL | 22 | |
| PLANTAR FASCIA ROLLING – BALL | 23 | |
| PLANTAR FASCIA ROLLING - COLD SODA CAN | 24 | |

# Myofascial Release

| _____ Reps _____ Sets _____ X Day _____ Hold | _____ Reps _____ Sets _____ X Day _____ Hold |
|---|---|
| **1** Notes: | **2** Notes: |

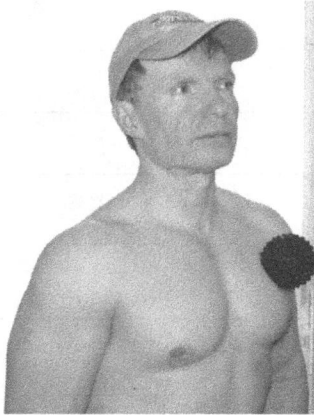

**ANTERIOR CHEST - BALL**

Face towards the wall and place small ball at the outside of chest. Bend knees up and down to find the target point and hold.

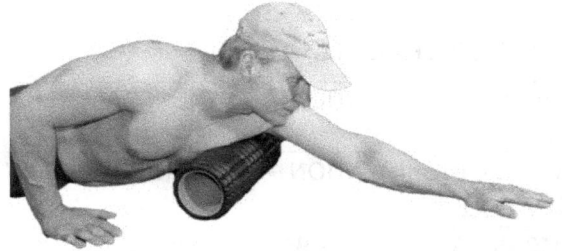

**ANTERIOR CHEST - FOAM ROLL**

Lie face down so that a foam roll is under the upper part of your arm and chest. Using your other arm and legs, roll forward and back across this area.

| _____ Reps _____ Sets _____ X Day _____ Hold | _____ Reps _____ Sets _____ X Day _____ Hold |
|---|---|
| **3** Notes: | **4** Notes: |

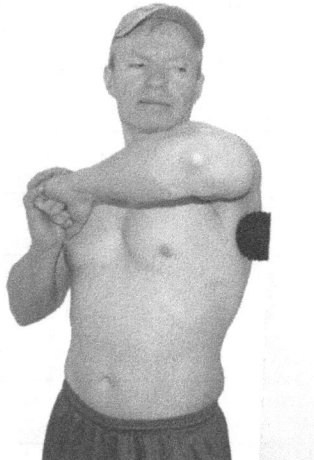

**LATISSIMUS DORSI – BALL**

Turn with your target side towards the wall and place small ball on the side under the shoulder. Bend knees up and down to find the target point and hold.

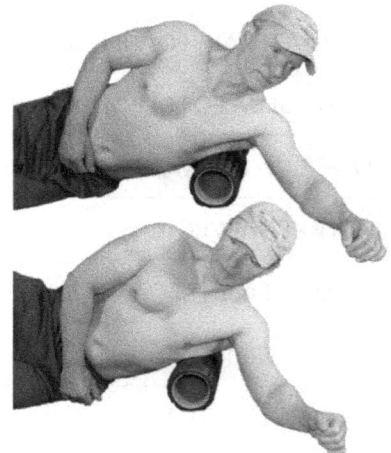

**LATISSIMUS DORSI - FOAM ROLL**

Lie on your side so that a foam roll is under the upper part of your arm and back. Using your other arm and legs, roll forward and back across this area.

| | |
|---|---|
| _____ Reps _____ Sets _____X Day _____Hold | _____ Reps _____ Sets _____X Day _____Hold |

**5** Notes:           **6** Notes:

TRICEP – FOAM ROLL

In a sidelying position, place your tricep on the foam roll. Use the opposite arm and your body to help roll out the arm on the foam roll.

OCCIPITAL RELEASE - FOAM ROLL

Lie on your back and put a foam roll under the back of your head. Turn your head slowly from side to side.

| | |
|---|---|
| _____ Reps _____ Sets _____X Day _____Hold | _____ Reps _____ Sets _____X Day _____Hold |

**7** Notes:           **8** Notes:

THORACIC MOBILIZATION – SUPINE - FOAM ROLL

Lie on a foam roller. While supporting your neck, roll up and down your mid-back.

THORACIC MOBILIZATION – STANDING - FOAM ROLL

Stand with a foam roll behind your upper back. Slowly perform mini-squats and allow the foam roller to roll up and down your back for a self-massage.

| | _____ Reps _____ Sets _____X Day _____Hold | | _____ Reps _____ Sets _____X Day _____Hold |
|---|---|---|---|
| **9** | Notes: | **10** | Notes: |

LUMBAR – STANDING – BALL - can do with foam roll

Place small ball in lower back on the side of the spine. DO NOT roll directly over the spine. Slowly perform mini-squats and allow the ball to roll up and down your back for a self-massage.
*Can use foam roll behind lower back and follow above directions.

LUMBAR – SUPINE – FOAM ROLLER

Lie on a foam roll under the lower back. While supporting your upper body, roll up and down your lower back.

| | _____ Reps _____ Sets _____X Day _____Hold | | _____ Reps _____ Sets _____X Day _____Hold |
|---|---|---|---|
| **11** | Notes: | **12** | Notes: |

↑
**Ball under hip flexor**

HIP FLEXORS - BALL

Lie on your stomach and place small ball under hip flexor. Roll up and down ball making small movements and hold on the target muscle.

HIP FLEXORS – FOAM ROLL

Lie on your stomach and place foam roll under both hip flexors. Roll up and down avoiding rolling directly over hip bones.

| | _____ Reps _____ Sets _____ X Day _____ Hold |
|---|---|
| **13** | **Notes:** |

QUADRICEPS – BILATERAL - FOAM ROLL

Lie face down so that a foam roll is under the top of your thighs. Using your arms propped on your elbows, roll forward and back across this area.

| | _____ Reps _____ Sets _____ X Day _____ Hold |
|---|---|
| **14** | **Notes:** |

QUADRICEP – SINGLE - FOAM ROLL

Lie face down so that a foam roll is under the top of your target thigh. Cross your other leg over the top of your target leg. Using your arms propped on your elbows, roll forward and back across this area.

| | _____ Reps _____ Sets _____ X Day _____ Hold |
|---|---|
| **15** | **Notes:** |

GLUTE /PIRIFORMIS - FOAM ROLL

Sit on a foam roll and cross your affected leg on top of your other knee. Lean slightly towards your target side. Using your arms and unaffected leg roll forward and back across your buttock area.

| | _____ Reps _____ Sets _____ X Day _____ Hold |
|---|---|
| **16** | **Notes:** |

HIP ADDUCTORS – FOAM ROLL

Lie on your stomach supported by arms and lace your inner thigh on the roller. Roll and compress the target thigh muscle.

| | _____ Reps _____ Sets _____X Day _____Hold |
|---|---|
| **17** | **Notes:** |

HAMSTRING – BILATERAL - FOAM ROLL

Sit on a foam roll under both thighs.  Using your arms, roll forward and back across this area

| | _____ Reps _____ Sets _____X Day _____Hold |
|---|---|
| **18** | **Notes:** |

HAMSTRING – SINGLE – FOAM ROLL

Sit on a foam roll under thigh.  Using your arms, roll forward and back across this area.

| | _____ Reps _____ Sets _____X Day _____Hold |
|---|---|
| **19** | **Notes:** |

CALVES – BILATERAL - FOAM ROLL

Sit with the foam roll under your both your calves. Lift your body up with your arms and roll forward and back across your calf area.  Try turning toes in and out to access the inside and outside of calf areas.  Do not roll in the crease of your knee.

| | _____ Reps _____ Sets _____X Day _____Hold |
|---|---|
| **20** | **Notes:** |

CALVES – SINGLE - FOAM ROLL

Sit with the foam roll under your target calf and cross your other leg on top. Lift your body up with your arms and roll forward and back across your calf area.  Do not roll in the crease of your knee.

|  | _____ Reps _____ Sets _____X Day _____Hold |
|---|---|
| **21** | **Notes:** |

ILIOTIBIAL BAND (IT Band) - FOAM ROLL

Lie on your side with a foam roll under your bottom thigh. Use your arms and unaffected leg and then roll up and down the foam roll along the outside of your thigh.

|  | _____ Reps _____ Sets _____X Day _____Hold |
|---|---|
| **22** | **Notes:** |

ILIOTIBIAL BAND (IT Band) - BALL

Lie on your side or sit in chair. Hold small ball and move along the outside of the thigh. Hold on the target muscle.

|  | _____ Reps _____ Sets _____X Day _____Hold |
|---|---|
| **23** | **Notes:** |

PLANTAR FASCIA ROLLING – BALL

Sit and place ball under foot. Roll plantar fascia over ball back and forth.

|  | _____ Reps _____ Sets _____X Day _____Hold |
|---|---|
| **24** | **Notes:** |

PLANTAR FASCIA ROLLING - COLD SODA CAN

Sit and place cold soda can under foot. Roll plantar fascia over can back and forth.

# Flexibility (Stretching)

Range of motion within a joint across various planes of motion that can be increased with stretching. This is needed to prevent decreased range of motion in a joint. Joint mobility can be inhibited by body habitués, genetics, connective tissue elasticity, skin that surrounds the joint, or the joint itself.

| | |
|---|---|
| **Some of the benefits of stretching:**<br><br>*(ACE Personal Training Manual)* | • Increased physical efficiency and performance.<br>• Decreased risk of injury by decreasing resistance in various tissues.<br>• Increased blood supply and nutrients to joint structures.<br>• Improved nutrient exchange by increasing the quantity and decreasing the thickness of synovial fluid in the joint.<br>• Increased neuromuscular coordination.<br>• Improved muscular balance and postural awareness.<br>• Reduced muscular tension. *(Bryant & Daniel, Ace Personal Training Manual, 2003, pg 306-307)* |
| **Things to remember when stretching** | • It is always better to stretch a warm muscle (*see Warm up and Cool down*) when the tissue temperature is above normal. Think of putting an elastic band in the freezer compared to heating it before stretching. Which do you think will get a better stretch?<br>• Static stretching is best for the type for beginning athletes. Static stretching is a slow, gradual lengthening of the connective tissue (tendon, muscles and ligaments) through a full range of motion to the point of discomfort – not pain. This stretch should be held for at least 30 seconds, but no longer than two minutes.<br>• Dynamic stretching consists of controlled leg and arm swings that take you to the limits of your range of motion. This type of stretching is appropriate to perform part of a warmup and/or cool down.<br>• Ballistic stretching is a rapid, bouncing movement that may be appropriate in some sports. The problem is that there is also a high-risk factor for injury and should only be done with a professional's guidance.<br>• Again, always remember to warm up before stretching. Repeat all stretches 2-3 times and hold for 15-30 seconds up to 60 seconds) unless otherwise indicated.<br>• Some evidence shows that static stretching may be more beneficial at the end of the exercise program when there is more certainty that the muscles have warmed up.<br>• Dynamic stretching may be more beneficial at the beginning of the exercise program as part of your warmup. This can also be done at the end as part of the cool down. |

| EXERCISE<br><br>Flexibility (Stretching) | EXERCISE NUMBER | NOTES |
|---|---|---|
| INVERSION | 1 | |
| EVERSION | 2 | |
| ANTERIOR TIBIALIS | 3 | |
| PLANTARFLEXION | 4 | |
| DORSIFLEXION - STRAP | 5 | |
| DORSIFLEXION - FLOOR ASSISTED | 6 | |
| STANDING CALF STRETCH - GASTROC | 7 | |
| STANDING CALF STRETCH - GASTROC – HAND ON KNEE | 8 | |
| GASTROCNEMIUS STAIR STRETCH | 9 | |
| STANDING CALF STRETCH - SOLEUS | 10 | |
| HAMSTRING STRETCH – TOWEL, BAND, STRAP or BELT | 11 | |
| HAMSTRING STRETCH – TOWEL, BAND, STRAP or BELT | 12 | |
| HAMSTRING STRETCH - TABLE, BED OR COUCH | 13 | |
| HAMSTRING / KNEE EXTENSION STRETCH - SEATED | 14 | |
| HAMSTRING STRETCH - STANDING | 15 | |
| TOE TOUCH – STANDING - NARROW or WIDE BOS | 16 | |
| HEEL SLIDES - SELF ASSISTED | 17 | |
| HEEL SLIDES - LONG SIT ASSISTED - TOWEL, BAND, STRAP or BELT | 18 | |
| HEEL SLIDES - SUPINE | 19 | |
| KNEE BENDS - EXERCISE BALL | 20 | |
| KNEE FLEXION – SELF ASSISTED - PRONE | 21 | |
| KNEE FLEXION – BELT ASSISTED - PRONE | 22 | |
| HEEL SLIDES - SELF ASSISTED | 23 | |
| HEEL SLIDES - SEATED | 24 | |
| KNEE FLEXION – SCOOT FORWARD - SEATED | 25 | |

| EXERCISE<br><br>**Flexibility (Stretching)** | EXERCISE NUMBER | NOTES |
|---|---|---|
| KNEE FLEXION – STAIR OR STEP | 26 | |
| PIRIFORMIS STRETCH | 27 | |
| PIRIFORMIS STRETCH - EXERCISE BALL | 28 | |
| PIRIFORMIS STRETCH - LONG SIT | 29 | |
| PIRIFORMIS STRETCH – STANDING | 30 | |
| HIP FLEXOR STRETCH - SIDE OF BALL or CHAIR | 31 | |
| HIP FLEXOR STRETCH - STANDING | 32 | |
| HIP FLEXOR STRETCH - HALF KNEEL | 33 | |
| RUNNER'S STRETCH - MODIFIED | 34 | |
| HIP FLEXOR STRETCH – SUPINE | 35 | |
| HIP FLEXOR STRETCH – SUPINE - 2 | 36 | |
| QUAD STRETCH - SIDELYING | 37 | |
| QUAD STRETCH - STANDING | 38 | |
| KNEE FALL OUT STRETCH or FROG STRETCH | 39 | |
| BUTTERFLY STRETCH | 40 | |
| HIP ADDUCTOR STRECH – KNEELING | 41 | |
| HIP ADDUCTOR STRECH - STANDING | 42 | |
| HIP EXTERNAL ROTATION STRETCH - SUPINE | 43 | |
| HIP INTERNAL ROTATION STRETCH - SEATED | 44 | |
| IT BAND STRETCH - STANDING | 45 | |
| IT BAND STRETCH -- SIDELYING | 46 | |
| NECK ROTATION and SIDE BENDS | 47 | |
| NECK FLEXION AND EXTENSION | 48 | |
| TRUNK FLEXION - SEATED | 49 | |
| LOW BACK STRETCH - SEATED | 50 | |
| LOW BACK STRETCH – STANDING - STRAIGHT & LATERAL | 51 | |
| LOW BACK STRETCH – RAIL OR DOORKNOB | 52 | |

| EXERCISE<br><br>Flexibility (Stretching) | EXERCISE NUMBER | NOTES |
|---|---|---|
| PRAYER STRETCH and LATERAL | 53 | |
| PRAYER STRETCH - EXERCISE BALL | 54 | |
| CAT AND CAMEL | 55 | |
| KNEE TO CHEST STRETCH - SINGLE and BILATERAL | 56 | |
| PRONE ON ELBOWS | 57 | |
| PRESS UPS | 58 | |
| TRUNK ROTATION STRETCH – SINGLE LEG | 59 | |
| LOWER TRUNK ROTATIONS – BILATERAL | 60 | |
| TRUNK ROTATION - SEATED | 61 | |
| TRUNK ROTATION - STANDING or SEATED – DOWEL | 62 | |
| LATERAL TRUNK STRETCH - SINGLE, SEATED or STANDING | 63 | |
| LATERAL TRUNK STRETCH - BILATERAL SEATED or STANDING | 64 | |
| FLEXION  - SUPINE - DOWEL | 65 | |
| WALL WALK | 66 | |
| FLEXION - TABLE SLIDE | 67 | |
| FLEXION - TABLE SLIDE -  BALL | 68 | |
| EXTERNAL ROTATION - SUPINE – DOWEL<br>*INTERNAL ROTATION ON OPPOSITE ARM* | 69 | |
| EXTERNAL ROTATION - 90-90 - DOWEL | 70 | |
| EXTERNAL ROTATION – SEATED – DOWEL<br>*INTERNAL ROTATION ON OPPOSITE ARM* | 71 | |
| EXTERNAL ROTATION – STANDING – DOWEL<br>*INTERNAL ROTATION ON OPPOSITE ARM* | 72 | |
| ABDUCTION - TABLE SLIDE - BALL | 75 | |
| ABDUCTION WITH DOWEL | 76 | |
| LYING DOWN EXTENSION - TABLE or BED | 77 | |
| WAND EXTENSION - STANDING | 78 | |
| CHEST STRETCH – SEATED,  STANDING, or SUPINE | 79 | |

**Flexibility (Stretching)**

| EXERCISE<br><br>Flexibility (Stretching) | EXERCISE NUMBER | NOTES |
|---|---|---|
| TRICEP STRETCH - STRAP or TOWEL | 82 | |
| POSTERIOR SHOULDER/DELTOID RELEASE | 83 | |
| POSTERIOR CAPSULE STRETCH | 84 | |

# Stretching / Range of Motion (ROM)

## Inversion

| _____ Reps | _____ Sets | _____ X Day | _____ Hold |

**1** | Notes:

INVERSION

Sit and cross your legs so that the target leg is on top. Hold your foot and pull upwards until a stretch is felt along the side of your ankle.

## Eversion

| _____ Reps | _____ Sets | _____ X Day | _____ Hold |

**2** | Notes:

EVERSION

Sit and cross your legs so that the target leg is on top. Hold your foot and push downward until a stretch is felt along the inner side of your ankle.

## Anterior  Tibialis (Ant Tib)

| _____ Reps | _____ Sets | _____ X Day | _____ Hold |

**3** | Notes:

ANTERIOR TIBIALIS

Kneel upright and slowly sit back onto legs forcing heels down towards floor. Sit back until stretch is felt.

## Plantarflexion  (PF)   *DF not shown*

| _____ Reps | _____ Sets | _____ X Day | _____ Hold |

**4** | Notes:

PLANTARFLEXION

Sit and place your affected foot on a firm surface. Use one hand bend the ankle downward as shown.

DORSIFLEXION – *Not shown*
Sit and place your affected foot on a firm surface. Use one hand under foot to push up towards shin (see #5 for movement)

## Dorsiflexion (DF)

| | _____ Reps _____ Sets _____ X Day _____ Hold | | _____ Reps _____ Sets _____ X Day _____ Hold |
|---|---|---|---|
| **5** | Notes: | **6** | Notes: |

**DORSIFLEXION - STRAP**

Sit with heel on floor and leg straight. Place belt/strap on forefoot and pull back until stretch is felt.

**DORSIFLEXION - FLOOR ASSISTED**

Sit and slide your foot back towards under the chair until a stretch is felt at the ankle.

## Gastroc/Soleus

| | _____ Reps _____ Sets _____ X Day _____ Hold | | _____ Reps _____ Sets _____ X Day _____ Hold |
|---|---|---|---|
| **7** | Notes: | **8** | Notes: |

Target Leg

**STANDING CALF STRETCH - GASTROC**

Stand in front of a wall, chair, or other sturdy object. Step forward with one foot and maintain your toes on both feet to be pointed straight forward. Keep the leg behind you with a straight knee during the stretch. Lean forward as you allow your front knee to bend until a stretch is felt along the back of your leg. Move closer or further away from the wall to control the stretch of the back leg.

Target Leg

**STANDING CALF STRETCH - GASTROC – HAND ON KNEE**

Step forward with one foot and place hand on thigh. Maintain your toes on both feet to be pointed straight forward. Keep the leg behind you with a straight knee during the stretch. Lean forward as you allow your front knee to bend until a stretch is felt along the back of your leg. You can adjust the bend of the front knee to control the stretch.

| | _____ Reps _____ Sets _____X Day _____Hold | | _____ Reps _____ Sets _____X Day _____Hold |
|---|---|---|---|
| **9** | **Notes:** | **10** | **Notes:** |

GASTROCNEMIUS STAIR STRETCH

Stand with the middle of your foot on the edge of the stairs while holding onto the railing. Slowly drop heels off until you feel a stretch in the back of your legs keeping your knees straight.

STANDING CALF STRETCH  - SOLEUS

Stand in front of a wall, chair or other sturdy object. Step forward with one foot and maintain your toes on both feet to be pointed straight forward. Keep the leg behind you with a slightly  bent knee during the stretch.  Lean forward towards the wall and support yourself with your arms as you allow your front knee to bend until a gentle stretch is felt along the back of your leg.  *Move closer or further away from the wall to control the stretch of the back leg. You can also adjust the bend of the front knee to control the stretch.

## Hamstring / Knee Extension

| | _____ Reps _____ Sets _____X Day _____Hold | | _____ Reps _____ Sets _____X Day _____Hold |
|---|---|---|---|
| **11** | **Notes:** | **12** | **Notes:** |

HAMSTRING STRETCH – TOWEL, BAND, STRAP or BELT

Lie down on your back and hook a towel/strap under your foot and draw up your leg until a stretch is felt under your leg/calf area.  Keep your knee in a straightened position during the stretch.  To increase stretch move strap to forefoot and flex foot.

HAMSTRING STRETCH – TOWEL, BAND, STRAP or BELT

While pushing down on thigh above knee cap with opposite hand, pull on towel/ strap to lift heel from floor. Keep thigh flat.  To increase stretch move strap to forefoot and flex foot and/or lean forward at the hip.

| _____ Reps _____ Sets _____ X Day _____ Hold | | _____ Reps _____ Sets _____ X Day _____ Hold |
|---|---|---|

**13** | Notes:

HAMSTRING STRETCH - TABLE, BED OR COUCH

Sit on a raised flat surface where you can prop your target leg up on it such as a treatment table, couch or bed.  While keeping your knee straight, slowly lean forward and reach your hands towards your foot until a gentle stretch is felt along the back of your knee/thigh. Hold and then return to starting position and repeat. Allow gravity to stretch your knee towards a more straightened position.
* Can use strap, towel or belt around forefoot as in #12

**14** | Notes:

HAMSTRING / KNEE EXTENSION STRETCH - SEATED

Sit and tighten your top thigh muscle to press the back of your knee downward towards the ground. You should feel a gentle stretch in the back of your knee.

* To increase stretch put strap to forefoot, flex foot and lean forward at the hip.

| _____ Reps _____ Sets _____ X Day _____ Hold | | _____ Reps _____ Sets _____ X Day _____ Hold |
|---|---|---|

**15** | Notes:

HAMSTRING STRETCH - STANDING

Stand and rest your foot on a stool/box/step with your knee straight. Gently lean forward at the hips until a stretch is felt behind your knee/thigh. Keep your back straight. *To increase stretch, flex your foot at the ankle, and/or put strap to forefoot and flex foot. If on stair, you can put foot on 2nd or 3rd step.

**16** | Notes:

TOE TOUCH – STANDING -  NARROW or WIDE BOS

Stand and bend forward at waist keep legs straight and reach for toes.  Can perform with either narrow or wide base of support.

## Knee Flexion

| | |
|---|---|
| _____ Reps _____ Sets _____X Day _____Hold | _____ Reps _____ Sets _____X Day _____Hold |

**17** Notes:

**18** Notes:

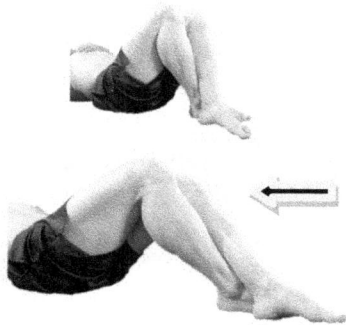

**HEEL SLIDES - SELF ASSISTED**

Lie on your back with knees straight and slide the target heel towards your buttock as you bend your knee. Use the unaffected leg to assist the bending. Hold a gentle stretch in this position and then return to original position.

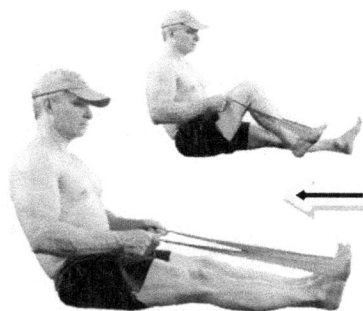

**HEEL SLIDES - LONG SIT ASSISTED - TOWEL, BAND, STRAP or BELT**

Sit with legs straight. Can place a small hand towel under your heel to help slide. Loop a band around your foot and pull your knee into a bend position as your foot slides towards your buttock. Hold a gentle stretch and then return back to original position.

| | |
|---|---|
| _____ Reps _____ Sets _____X Day _____Hold | _____ Reps _____ Sets _____X Day _____Hold |

**19** Notes:

**20** Notes:

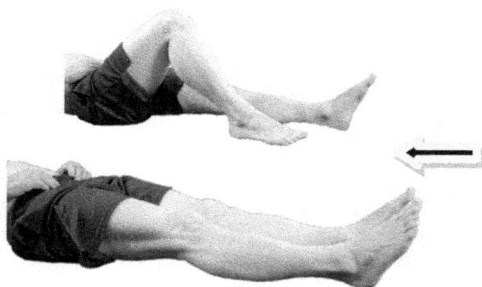

**HEEL SLIDES - SUPINE**

Lie on your back with knees straight and slide the target heel towards your buttock as you bend your knee. Hold a gentle stretch in this position and then return to original position.

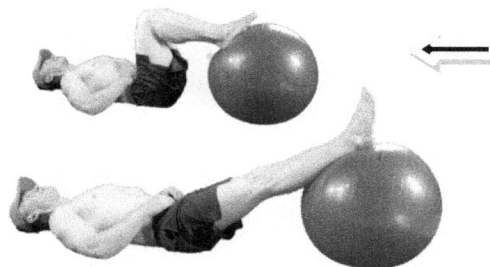

**KNEE BENDS - EXERCISE BALL**

Lie on your back and place your heels on an exercise ball. Roll it closer to your buttocks as your knees and hips bend as shown. Hold and then return to original position. *If you have limited range in one knee, use the other leg to help increase range of motion.

## Flexibility (Stretching)

| | |
|---|---|
| _____ Reps _____ Sets _____ X Day _____ Hold | _____ Reps _____ Sets _____ X Day _____ Hold |
| **21** Notes: | **22** Notes: |

KNEE FLEXION – SELF ASSISTED - PRONE

Lie face down and bend your target knee with the assistance of your unaffected leg.

KNEE FLEXION – BELT ASSISTED - PRONE

Lie face down with a strap looped around your target side ankle or foot. Use the belt to pull the knee into a bent position allowing for a stretch.

| | |
|---|---|
| _____ Reps _____ Sets _____ X Day _____ Hold | _____ Reps _____ Sets _____ X Day _____ Hold |
| **23** Notes: | **24** Notes: |

HEEL SLIDES - SELF ASSISTED

It and slide your heel towards your buttock with the assist of the unaffected leg. Hold a gentle stretch and then return foot forward to original position.

HEEL SLIDES - SEATED – can use towel or paper under foot to help slide

Sit and place your feet on the floor (can put target foot on a towel or paper to help slide if needed). Slowly slide your foot closer towards you. Hold a gentle stretch and then return foot forward to original position.

| _____ Reps _____ Sets _____X Day _____Hold | _____ Reps _____ Sets _____X Day _____Hold |
|---|---|
| **25** Notes: | **26** Notes: |

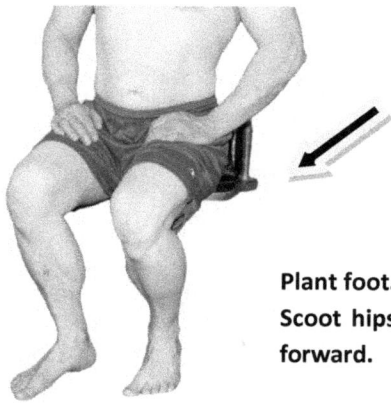

Plant foot.
Scoot hips
forward.

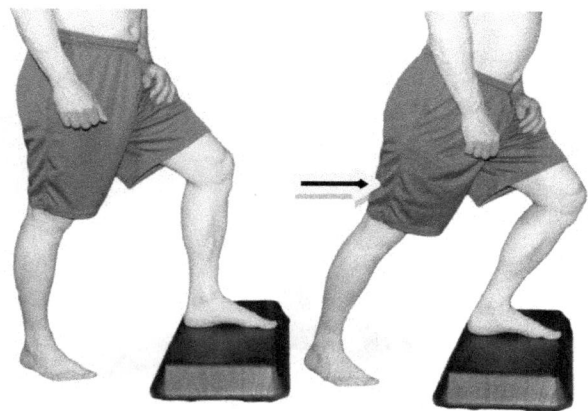

KNEE FLEXION – SCOOT FORWARD - SEATED

Sit and slide your foot back to a bent knee position. Keep your foot planted on the ground and scoot forward until a stretch is felt at the knee.  Hold the stretch and then scoot back to original position.

KNEE FLEXION – STAIR OR STEP

Place target foot on stool or step with bent knee. Gently bend forward keeping heel on step.  Hold the stretch and then return to original position.

## Piriformis

| _____ Reps _____ Sets _____X Day _____Hold | _____ Reps _____ Sets _____X Day _____Hold |
|---|---|
| **27** Notes: | **28** Notes: |

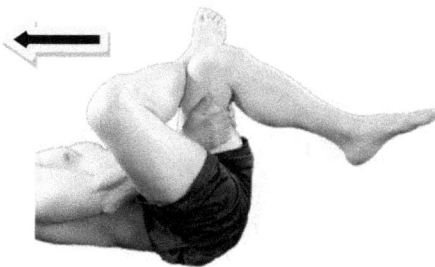

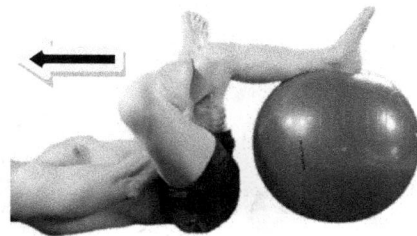

PIRIFORMIS STRETCH

Lie on your back with both knees bent.  Cross your target leg on the other knee.  Hold your unaffected thigh and pull it up towards your chest until a stretch is felt in the buttock.

PIRIFORMIS STRETCH - EXERCISE BALL

Lie on your back with one foot placed on the ball. Cross your other leg over the knee of the leg on the ball and gently roll the ball back towards your chest until a stretch is felt in the buttock.

| | \_\_\_\_\_ Reps \_\_\_\_\_ Sets \_\_\_\_\_X Day \_\_\_\_\_Hold | | \_\_\_\_\_ Reps \_\_\_\_\_ Sets \_\_\_\_\_X Day \_\_\_\_\_Hold |
|---|---|---|---|
| **29** | Notes: | **30** | Notes: |

**PIRIFORMIS STRETCH - LONG SIT**

Sit with one knee straight and the other bent and placed over the opposite knee. Gentle turn your body towards the bend knee side.

**PIRIFORMIS STRETCH – STANDING**

Stand with unaffected leg crossed in front of target side. Lean forward reaching for foot on target side until stretch is felt in the buttock.

## Hip Flexors

| | \_\_\_\_\_ Reps \_\_\_\_\_ Sets \_\_\_\_\_X Day \_\_\_\_\_Hold | | \_\_\_\_\_ Reps \_\_\_\_\_ Sets \_\_\_\_\_X Day \_\_\_\_\_Hold |
|---|---|---|---|
| **31** | Notes: | **32** | Notes: |

**HIP FLEXOR STRETCH - SIDE OF BALL or CHAIR**

Sit on edge of chair or ball. Bend your front knee (unaffected side) and lean forward until a stretch is felt along the front of the target hip.

**HIP FLEXOR STRETCH - STANDING**

Stand and bend one knee forward (unaffected side) and the other in back. Stand up straight leaning slightly backward until a stretch is felt along the front of the target hip.

| | _____ Reps _____ Sets _____ X Day _____ Hold |
|---|---|
| **33** | **Notes:** |

HIP FLEXOR STRETCH - HALF KNEEL – with or without pad under knee

Begin in a half-kneeling position (you may want to use a pad or pillow for cushion). Bend your front knee (unaffected side) and lean forward until a stretch is felt along the front of the target hip.

| | _____ Reps _____ Sets _____ X Day _____ Hold |
|---|---|
| **34** | **Notes:** |

RUNNER'S STRETCH - MODIFIED

Stretch target leg in back and bend other knee in front. Bend your front knee (unaffected side) and lean forward until a stretch is felt along the front of the target hip.

| | _____ Reps _____ Sets _____ X Day _____ Hold |
|---|---|
| **35** | **Notes:** |

HIP FLEXOR STRETCH – SUPINE

Lie on a table, high bed or matt and let the affected leg lower towards the floor until a stretch is felt along the front of your thigh.

| | _____ Reps _____ Sets _____ X Day _____ Hold |
|---|---|
| **36** | **Notes:** |

HIP FLEXOR STRETCH – SUPINE

Lie on a table, high bed or matt and let the affected leg lower towards the floor until a stretch is felt along the front of your thigh. At the same time, grasp your opposite knee and pull it towards your chest.

## Quadriceps (Quad)

| | \_\_\_\_\_ Reps \_\_\_\_\_ Sets \_\_\_\_\_X Day \_\_\_\_\_Hold | | \_\_\_\_\_ Reps \_\_\_\_\_ Sets \_\_\_\_\_X Day \_\_\_\_\_Hold |
|---|---|---|---|
| **37** | Notes: | **38** | Notes: |

QUAD STRETCH - SIDELYING

Lie on your side and reach back holding the top of your foot with bent knee until a stretch is felt.

QUAD STRETCH - STANDING

Stand straight up and bend your knee in back holding your ankle/foot. Gently pull your knee/thigh back in alignment with the standing leg.

## Adductor

| | \_\_\_\_\_ Reps \_\_\_\_\_ Sets \_\_\_\_\_X Day \_\_\_\_\_Hold | | \_\_\_\_\_ Reps \_\_\_\_\_ Sets \_\_\_\_\_X Day \_\_\_\_\_Hold |
|---|---|---|---|
| **39** | Notes: | **40** | Notes: |

One Leg

Both Legs

KNEE FALL OUT STRETCH or FROG STRETCH

Lie on your back with one knee bent. Slowly lower your knee to the side as you stretch the inner thigh/hip area. Frog Stretch: Let both knees fall to the side at the same time.

BUTTERFLY STRETCH

Sit on the floor or mat and bend your knees placing the bottom of your feet together. Slowly let your knees lower towards the floor until a stretch is felt at your inner thighs.

| | _____ Reps _____ Sets _____X Day _____Hold | | _____ Reps _____ Sets _____X Day _____Hold |
|---|---|---|---|
| **41** | **Notes:** | **42** | **Notes:** |

Target Leg

HIP ADDUCTOR STRECH – KNEELING

Kneel down on your target side knee. Place the opposite leg directly out to the side. Lean towards the side as you bend the knee for a stretch to the inner thigh of the target leg.

Target Leg

HIP ADDUCTOR STRECH - STANDING

Stand with feet spread wide apart. Slowly bend your knee to allow for a gentle stretch of the opposite leg. Maintain a straight knee on the target leg the entire time. You should feel a stretch on the inner thigh.

## External Rotation / Internal Rotation

| | _____ Reps _____ Sets _____X Day _____Hold | | _____ Reps _____ Sets _____X Day _____Hold |
|---|---|---|---|
| **43** | **Notes:** | **44** | **Notes:** |

HIP EXTERNAL ROTATION STRETCH - SUPINE

Lie on your back with your leg crossed over your knee. Use your hand and push the crossed knee away from you.

HIP INTERNAL ROTATION STRETCH  - SEATED

Sit on a chair with your legs spread apart and feet planted on the ground.  Use your hand to draw your knee inward as shown.

# Iliotibial Band (IT Band)

| | |
|---|---|
| _____ Reps _____ Sets _____ X Day _____ Hold | _____ Reps _____ Sets _____ X Day _____ Hold |
| **45** Notes: | **46** Notes: |

IT BAND STRETCH - STANDING

Stand and cross the target leg behind your unaffected leg. Lean forward and towards the unaffected side while using your arm for balance support.

IT BAND STRETCH -- SIDELYING

Lie on bed or couch on unaffected side with target side towards ceiling. Bend lower leg for support. Allow upper leg to drop over side of bed. Keep knee straight and point toe towards floor. May need to roll upper hip backwards in order to feel stretch on side of hip/thigh/knee.

# NECK

| | |
|---|---|
| _____ Reps _____ Sets _____ X Day _____ Hold | _____ Reps _____ Sets _____ X Day _____ Hold |
| **47** Notes: | **48** Notes: |

NECK ROTATION and SIDE BENDS

SIDE BENDS: (*Top*) Tilt your head as if you are trying to touch your ear to your shoulder. For extra stretch gently use your hand to increase range and hold.
ROTATION: (*Bottom*) Turn your head to the side as if looking over your shoulder. For an extra stretch gently use your hand on your chin to increase range and hold.

NECK FLEXION AND EXTENSION

EXTENSION: Look up as if you are looking at the sky moving your neck only.
FLEXION: Look down as if you are looking at the floor. For an extra stretch gently put both hands behind your head to move chin towards the chest and hold.

## BACK

| _____ Reps _____ Sets _____ X Day _____ Hold | | _____ Reps _____ Sets _____ X Day _____ Hold | |
|---|---|---|---|
| **49** | Notes: | **50** | Notes: |

TRUNK FLEXION - SEATED

Sit and cross your arms over your chest. Slowly curl your back forward in order to round your upper back.

LOW BACK STRETCH - SEATED

Sit and slowly bend forward reaching your hands for the floor. Bend your trunk and head forward and down.

| _____ Reps _____ Sets _____ X Day _____ Hold | | _____ Reps _____ Sets _____ X Day _____ Hold | |
|---|---|---|---|
| **51** | Notes: | **52** | Notes: |

LOW BACK STRETCH – STANDING - STRAIGHT & LATERAL

Stand in front of a table / chair or other surface and bend forward at the waist. Support yourself with your hands on a surface.

Reach to the side for a lateral bend (see #53)

LOW BACK STRETCH – RAIL OR DOORKNOB

Hold onto doorknob, rail or other unmovable surface and pull while moving hips back and hold.

# Flexibility (Stretching)

| _____ Reps _____ Sets _____X Day _____Hold | |
|---|---|
| **53** | **Notes:** |

Lateral

Straight

**PRAYER STRETCH and LATERAL**

STRAIGHT: Start on your hands and knees. Slowly lower your buttocks towards your feet until a stretch is felt along your back and or buttocks.

LATERAL: Start on your hands and knees. Slowly lower your buttocks towards your feet. Lower your chest towards the floor as you reach out towards the side.

| _____ Reps _____ Sets _____X Day _____Hold | |
|---|---|
| **54** | **Notes:** |

**PRAYER STRETCH - EXERCISE BALL**

Kneel with an exercise ball in front of you. Slowly lean forward and roll the ball forward until a stretch is felt.

*Can do lateral movement as in #53

| _____ Reps _____ Sets _____X Day _____Hold | |
|---|---|
| **55** | **Notes:** |

**CAT AND CAMEL**

Start on your hands and knees. Raise up your back and arch it towards the ceiling (cat). Return to a lowered position and arch your back the opposite direction (camel).

| _____ Reps _____ Sets _____X Day _____Hold | |
|---|---|
| **56** | **Notes:** |

Both Legs

One Leg

**KNEE TO CHEST STRETCH - SINGLE and BILATERAL**

BILATERAL: Lie on your back and hold your knees while pulling up towards your chest and hold.
SINGLE: Lie on your back and hold your knee while pulling up towards your chest and hold. Opposite leg can be straight or bent.

## Trunk Extension

| _____ Reps _____ Sets _____ X Day _____ Hold | | _____ Reps _____ Sets _____ X Day _____ Hold | |
|---|---|---|---|
| **57** | Notes: | **58** | Notes: |

PRONE ON ELBOWS

Lie on your stomach.  Slowly press up and prop yourself up on your elbows. Keep hips on floor/mat.

PRESS UPS

Lie on your stomach.  Slowly press up and arch your back using your arms.  Keep hips on floor/mat.

## Trunk Rotation

| _____ Reps _____ Sets _____ X Day _____ Hold | | _____ Reps _____ Sets _____ X Day _____ Hold | |
|---|---|---|---|
| **59** | Notes: | **60** | Notes: |

TRUNK ROTATION STRETCH – SINGLE LEG

Lie on your back with arms to the sides. Bend one knee and then raise it up and across your body. Allow your trunk to rotate for a gentle stretch to the spine. Hold and then repeat.

LOWER TRUNK ROTATIONS – BILATERAL

Lie on your back with your knees bent and gently move your knees side-to-side.

| | \_\_\_\_\_ Reps \_\_\_\_\_ Sets \_\_\_\_\_X Day \_\_\_\_\_Hold | | \_\_\_\_\_ Reps \_\_\_\_\_ Sets \_\_\_\_\_X Day \_\_\_\_\_Hold |
|---|---|---|---|
| **61** | Notes: | **62** | Notes: |

TRUNK ROTATION - SEATED

Sit up as tall with erect posture. Rotate in one direction, using your hand to press against the opposite thigh to aide in further rotation. Exhale to increase the rotation and stretch. Return to the starting position, maintain an upright posture -repeat in the opposite direction.

TRUNK ROTATION - STANDING or SEATED – DOWEL

Stand or sit holding dowel in hands. Slowly rotate trunk in one direction and then in the opposite direction.

## Lateral

| | \_\_\_\_\_ Reps \_\_\_\_\_ Sets \_\_\_\_\_X Day \_\_\_\_\_Hold | | \_\_\_\_\_ Reps \_\_\_\_\_ Sets \_\_\_\_\_X Day \_\_\_\_\_Hold |
|---|---|---|---|
| **63** | Notes: | **64** | Notes: |

LATERAL TRUNK STRETCH - SINGLE
SEATED or STANDING

Raise your arm and bend to the opposite side for a stretch. Hold and repeat with opposite arm.

LATERAL TRUNK STRETCH - BILATERAL
SEATED or STANDING

Clasp hands together and raise arms over head. Bend to one side. Hold and repeat in opposite direction.

## Shoulder Flexion

| | _____ Reps _____ Sets _____X Day _____Hold |
|---|---|
| **65** | **Notes:** |

FLEXION - SUPINE - DOWEL

Lie on your back and hold a dowel/cane. Slowly raise the dowel overhead.

*If you have a weak or injured arm, you can use your unaffected arm to assist with the movement.

| | _____ Reps _____ Sets _____X Day _____Hold |
|---|---|
| **66** | **Notes:** |

WALL WALK

Place your target hand on the wall with the palm facing the wall. Walk your fingers up the wall towards overhead. Slide or walk your hand back down the wall to the starting position.

| | _____ Reps _____ Sets _____X Day _____Hold |
|---|---|
| **67** | **Notes:** |

FLEXION - TABLE SLIDE

Sit or stand and rest your target arm on a table and gently slide it forward and then back.

| | _____ Reps _____ Sets _____X Day _____Hold |
|---|---|
| **68** | **Notes:** |

FLEXION - TABLE SLIDE - BALL

Stand and rest your target arm on top of a ball on a table. Gently roll the ball forward and then back.

**Flexibility (Stretching)**

## Shoulder External Rotation (ER)

| _____ Reps _____ Sets _____X Day _____Hold | | _____ Reps _____ Sets _____X Day _____Hold |
|---|---|---|

**69** Notes:

**70** Notes:

Starting
Position

EXTERNAL ROTATION - SUPINE – DOWEL
*INTERNAL ROTATION ON OPPOSITE ARM*

Lie on your back holding a dowel/cane with both hands. On the target side, maintain approx. 90-degree bend at the elbow with your arm approximately 30-45 degrees away from your side. Use your other arm to push the dowel/cane to rotate the affected arm back into a stretch. Hold and then return to starting position. Repeat

EXTERNAL ROTATION - 90-90 - DOWEL

Lie on your back and hold a dowel with your elbows out to the side and rested down. Roll your arms back towards overhead until a stretch is felt. Keep elbows bent at a 90-degree angle.

| _____ Reps _____ Sets _____X Day _____Hold | | _____ Reps _____ Sets _____X Day _____Hold |
|---|---|---|

**71** Notes:

**72** Notes:

EXTERNAL ROTATION – SEATED – DOWEL
*INTERNAL ROTATION ON OPPOSITE ARM*

Using the unaffected arm, push the dowel into the hand of the target arm. Keep the arm at a 90-degree angle and push until a stretch is felt. Hold and repeat.

EXTERNAL ROTATION – STANDING – DOWEL
*INTERNAL ROTATION ON OPPOSITE ARM*

Using the unaffected arm, push the dowel into the hand of the target arm. Keep the arm at a 90-degree angle and push until a stretch is felt. Hold and repeat.

## Shoulder Internal Rotation (IR) - *also see #69, 71, 72*

| | | |
|---|---|---|
| **73** | _____ Reps _____ Sets _____X Day _____Hold | |
| | **Notes:** | |

| | | |
|---|---|---|
| **74** | _____ Reps _____ Sets _____X Day _____Hold | |
| | **Notes:** | |

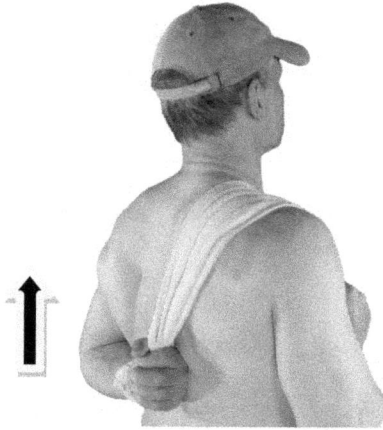

INTERNAL ROTATION – TOWEL OR STRAP

Hold one end of the towel in front and with the target arm behind your back. Gently pull up your target arm behind your back with the assist of a towel.

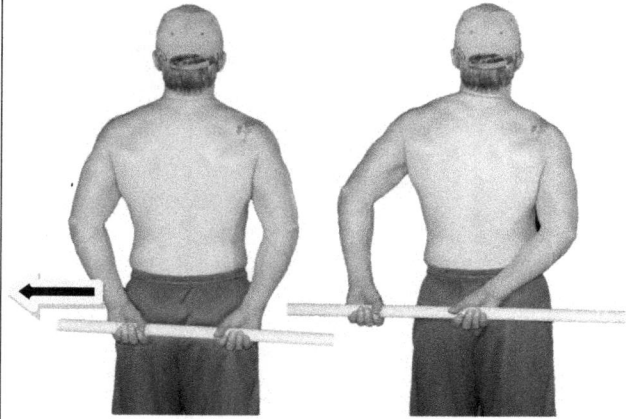

INTERNAL ROTATION – DOWEL

Hold a dowel/cane behind your back. Slowly pull the target arm towards the center of your back.

## Shoulder Abduction

| | | |
|---|---|---|
| **75** | _____ Reps _____ Sets _____X Day _____Hold | |
| | **Notes:** | |

| | | |
|---|---|---|
| **76** | _____ Reps _____ Sets _____X Day _____Hold | |
| | **Notes:** | |

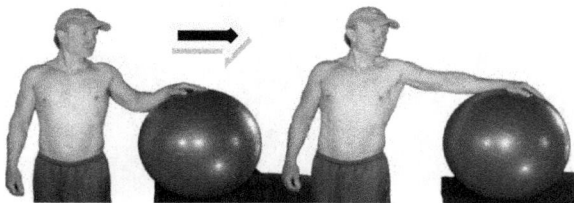

ABDUCTION - TABLE SLIDE - BALL

Stand and rest your target arm on top of a ball on a table and gently roll it to the side and back.

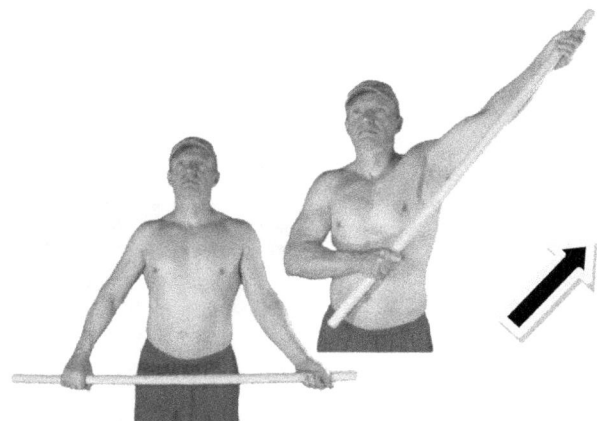

ABDUCTION WITH DOWEL

Hold a dowel/cane in front. Slowly push the dowel of the unaffected arm towards the target arm upward and to the side.

## Shoulder Extension

| | _____ Reps _____ Sets _____X Day _____Hold | | _____ Reps _____ Sets _____X Day _____Hold |
|---|---|---|---|
| **77** | Notes: | **78** | Notes: |

LYING DOWN EXTENSION - TABLE or BED

Lie on your back and gently let target arm drop off table or bed.

WAND EXTENSION - STANDING

Stand and hold a dowel/cane. Use the unaffected arm to help push the target arm back. The elbow should remain straight the entire time.

## Chest/Pec Stretch

| | _____ Reps _____ Sets _____X Day _____Hold | | _____ Reps _____ Sets _____X Day _____Hold |
|---|---|---|---|
| **79** | Notes: | **80** | Notes: |

CHEST STRETCH – SEATED, STANDING, or SUPINE

TOP: Bend arms at a 90-degree angle. Move elbows back until feeling a stretch in front of shoulders/chest.

BOTTOM: Clasp hands in back of head. Move elbows back until feeling a stretch in front of shoulders/chest.

CHEST STRETCH - STEP THROUGH

Stand with arms in doorway at a 90-degree angle. Step through until you feel a stretch through the chest and hold. Keep shoulders down and back. Take another step to increase stretch.

# Triceps

| | | | | | | |
|---|---|---|---|---|---|---|
| _____ Reps | _____ Sets | _____ X Day | _____ Hold | | | |

**81** Notes:

**TRICEP STRETCH**

With your target elbow bent and shoulder raised, use your other hand and gently push your target elbow back towards overhead until a stretch is felt.

| | | | |
|---|---|---|---|
| _____ Reps | _____ Sets | _____ X Day | _____ Hold |

**82** Notes:

**TRICEP STRETCH -  STRAP or TOWEL**

Hold strap of target arm with your hand above your head. Use the other hand to pull downward on the strap, allowing the elbow to bend until a stretch is in the back of the arm.

# Posterior Capsule

**83** Notes:

_____ Reps _____ Sets _____ X Day _____ Hold

**POSTERIOR SHOULDER/DELTOID RELEASE**

Bring your target arm across your body. Use the opposite hand to grasp the back of your shoulder and further pull the arm.  Hold.

**84** Notes:

_____ Reps _____ Sets _____ X Day _____ Hold

**POSTERIOR CAPSULE STRETCH**

Lie on your side and grasp the elbow of the arm closest to the floor.  Gently pull it upward and across the front of your body.

# Core / Stability Training

Core strengthening is the foundation of all the other exercises that follow, especially balance. Core training is not only an important step in conditioning, but also helps other issues, including neurological, orthopedic, weight, or overall weakness

The core includes muscles of the thoraco-lumbar spine (trunk), cervical spine., erector spinae, abdomen, pelvis, shoulder/scapulae, and your lower lats.

Static core functionality is the ability of one's core to align the skeleton to resist a force that does not change. The core is used to stabilize the thorax and the pelvis during dynamic movement. The nature of dynamic movement must consider our skeletal structure (as a lever) in addition to the force of external resistance and consequently incorporates a vastly different complex of muscles and joints versus a static position.

The core is traditionally assumed to originate most full-body functional movement, including most sports. In addition, the core determines to a large part a person's posture. In all, human anatomy is built to take force upon the bones and direct autonomic force, through various joints, in the desired direction. The core muscles align the spine, ribs, and pelvis of a person to resist a specific force, whether static or dynamic.
(Wikipedia: *https://en.wikipedia.org/wiki/Core_(anatomy)*

These muscles work as stabilizers for the entire body. Core training is simply doing specific exercises to develop and strengthen these stabilizer muscles. If any of these core muscles are weakened, it could result in lower back pain or a protruding waistline. Keeping these core muscles strong can do wonders for your posture and help give you more strength in other exercises like running and walking.
(Bodybuilding.com - *https://www.bodybuilding.com/fun/mielke12.htm*)

There is a saying 'form follows function'. This is especially true with core stability and how it affects your balance. Gravity influences all movement, so effective core training must be done against gravity. The rectus abdominus muscle that you are isolating with those crunches flexes the spine/abs only when you are lying on your back or returning the torso to an upright position from hyperextension in standing. "In the upright position, flexion is controlled by eccentric contraction of the back extensors as the lower the weight of the torso in the same direction as gravity". (*Bryant & Green, 2003, p. 84*)

Being able to engage the core with not only your balance exercises but also arm and leg exercises will help prevent injury.

Step 1: First learn to brace the abdomen *(see pictures 1 and 2 on next page)* Think of this as trying to either brace for a punch to the stomach or trying to put on a tight pair of pants (not just sucking in your stomach)

Step 2: After getting a good feel for bracing, try doing a pelvic tilt *(see pictures 3 and 4 on next page)* and then progress to bridging *(see picture 5)*

Step 3: These two basic movements should be done while you progress your abdominal and core training, continuing through the balance section, and to some extent with arm and leg strengthening.

*** **When doing floor work, such as crunches, make sure you are on a soft surface, such as a mat, Bosu, stability ball, etc. Pushing your back into a hard surface, such as a wood floor, can do more damage than good to the spine.**

*** **Breathe – Never hold your breath.**

## Core / Stability

| EXERCISE | EXERCISE NUMBER | NOTES |
| --- | --- | --- |
| Core / Stability | | |
| ABDOMINAL BRACING TRAINING | 1 | |
| ABDOMINAL BRACING - SUPINE | 2 | |
| PELVIC TILT - SUPINE | 3 | |
| PELVIC TILT - KNEELING | 4 | |
| BRIDGING | 5 | |
| BRIDGE - BOSU | 6 | |
| BRIDGING WITH PILLOW SQUEEZE | 7 | |
| BRIDGING WITH PILLOW SQUEEZE - BOSU | 8 | |
| BRACE SUPINE MARCHING / BRIDGE LEG UP | 9 | |
| BRIDGE LEG UP - BOSU - | 10 | |
| SINGLE LEG BRIDGE | 11 | |
| BRIDGE SINGLE LEG - BOSU | 12 | |
| BRIDGING CROSSED LEG | 13 | |
| BRIDGING CROSSED LEG – BOSU | 14 | |
| BRIDGING CROSSED LEG - ARMS UP | 15 | |
| BRIDGING CROSSED LEG - ARMS UP - BOSU | 16 | |
| BRIDGE - ELASTIC BAND | 17 | |
| BRIDGING - ABDUCTION - ELASTIC BAND | 18 | |
| FLOOR BRIDGE - EXERCISE BALL | 19 | |
| FLOOR BRIDGE ALTERNATE LEG LIFT - EXERCISE BALL | 20 | |
| BRIDGE UPPER BACK - EXERCISE BALL | 21 | |
| BRIDGE UPPER BACK - SINGLE LEG - EXERCISE BALL | 22 | |
| QUADRUPED ALTERNATE ARM | 23 | |
| QUADRUPED ALTERNATE LEG | 24 | |
| QUADRUPED ALTERNATE ARM AND LEG | 25 | |
| BIRD DOG ELBOW TOUCHES | 26 | |

| EXERCISE<br>Core / Stability | EXERCISE NUMBER | NOTES |
|---|---|---|
| PRONE BALL | 27 | |
| PRONE BALL - ALTERNATE ARM | 28 | |
| PRONE BALL - ALTERNATE LEG | 29 | |
| PRONE BALL - ALTERNATE ARM AND LEG | 30 | |
| MODIFIED PLANK | 31 | |
| MODIFIED PLANK - ALTERNATE LEG | 32 | |
| FULL PLANK | 33 | |
| PLANK - ALTERNATE ARMS | 34 | |
| PLANK - ALTERNATE LEGS | 35 | |
| PLANK - EXERCISE BALL | 36 | |
| PRONE ON ELBOWS | 37 | |
| PRESS UPS | 38 | |
| SKYDIVER | 39 | |
| PRONE SUPERMAN - BOSU | 40 | |
| TRUNK EXTENSION - BOSU | 41 | |
| TRUNK EXTENSION - HANDS CROSSED IN FRONT - BOSU | 43 | |
| SUPERMAN - ARMS BACK- EXERCISE BALL | 44 | |
| SUPERMAN – BOTH ARMS IN FRONT - EXERCISE BALL | 45 | |
| SUPERMAN – ONE ARM FORWARD / ONE ARM BACK - EXERCISE BALL | 46 | |
| LATERAL PLANK MODIFIED | 47 | |
| LATERAL PLANK MODIFIED- BOSU | 48 | |
| LATERAL PLANK - 1 KNEE 1 FOOT | 49 | |
| LATERAL PLANK - 1 KNEE 1 FOOT – BOSU | 50 | |
| LATERAL PLANK | 51 | |
| LATERAL PLANK - BOSU | 52 | |

| EXERCISE | EXERCISE NUMBER | NOTES |
|---|---|---|
| **Core / Stability** | | |
| LEAN BACK | 53 | |
| LEAN BACK - BOSU | 54 | |
| LEAN BACK WITH ARMS OUT | 55 | |
| LEAN BACK WITH ARMS OUT - BOSU | 56 | |
| LEAN BACK WITH TWIST | 57 | |
| LEAN BACK WITH TWIST – BOSU | 58 | |
| CRUNCHY FROG | 59 | |
| SEATED BIKE - FORWARD AND BACKWARDS | 60 | |
| CRUNCH – ARMS OUT | 61 | |
| CRUNCH – ARMS OUT - BOSU | 62 | |
| CRUNCH – ARMS IN BACK OF HEAD | 63 | |
| CRUNCH – ARMS IN BACK OF HEAD - BOSU | 64 | |
| OBLIQUE CRUNCH | 65 | |
| OBLIQUE CRUNCH - BOSU | 66 | |
| 90 DEGREE CRUNCH | 67 | |
| BALL CRUNCH – Can put legs on seat of chair | 68 | |
| CURL UPS – ARMS ON LEGS - EXERCISE BALL | 69 | |
| CURL UPS- ARMS CROSSED IN FRONT - EXERCISE BALL | 70 | |
| CURL UPS – ARMS BEHIND HEAD - EXERCISE BALL | 71 | |
| SUPINE CRUNCH TOUCH - EXERCISE BALL | 72 | |
| LOWER ABDOMINAL CRUNCH – WITH or WITHOUT BALL | 73 | |
| HIGH MARCH CRUNCH | 74 | |
| STANDING SIDE CRUNCH | 75 | |
| STANDING BIKE CRUNCH | 76 | |

# Core/Abdominal

## Abdominal Bracing – Pelvic Tilt

| | _____ Reps _____ Sets _____X Day _____Hold | | _____ Reps _____ Sets _____X Day _____Hold |
|---|---|---|---|
| **1** | Notes: | **2** | Notes: |

ABDOMINAL BRACING TRAINING

Press your fingertips into your relaxed abdomen lateral of your navel. Tighten and brace your abdomen so that the muscles push your fingertips away from the center of your body. Hold, relax and repeat.
_Think of this as trying to either brace for a punch to the stomach or trying to put on a tight pair of pants (not just sucking in your stomach)_

Starting Position

ABDOMINAL BRACING - SUPINE

Lie on your back. Tighten your stomach muscles as you draw your navel down towards the floor.

_Think of this as trying to either brace for a punch to the stomach or trying to put on a tight pair of pants (not just sucking in your stomach)_

| | _____ Reps _____ Sets _____X Day _____Hold | | _____ Reps _____ Sets _____X Day _____Hold |
|---|---|---|---|
| **3** | Notes: | **4** | Notes: |

Starting Position

PELVIC TILT - SUPINE

Lie on your back with your knees bent. Next, arch your low back and then flatten it repeatedly (bracing as above). Your pelvis should tilt forward and back during the movement. Move through a comfortable range of motion.

Starting Position

PELVIC TILT - KNEELING

Kneel on the floor (you can kneel on a pillow or pad if needed). Arch your lower back and then flatten it repeatedly (bracing as above). Your pelvis should tilt forward and back during the movement. Move through a comfortable range of motion.

# Bridging

| | _____ Reps _____ Sets _____X Day _____Hold | | _____ Reps _____ Sets _____X Day _____Hold |
|---|---|---|---|
| **5** | **Notes:** | **6** | **Notes:** |

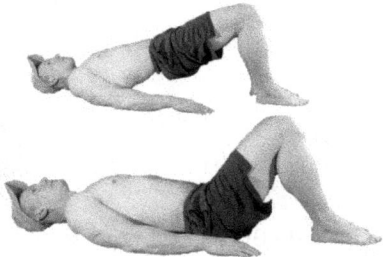

Starting

Position

BRIDGING

Lie on your back. Tighten your lower abdominals (as with abdominal bracing), squeeze your buttocks and then raise your buttocks off the floor/bed. Hold and then lower yourself slowly and repeat. Brace the stomach muscles to keep your spine from moving, trying to keep the pelvis level the entire time.

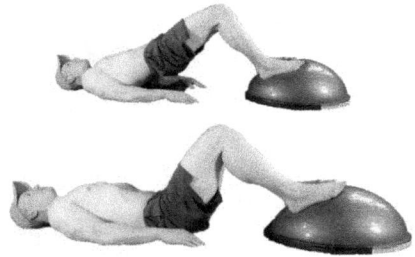

Starting
Position

BRIDGE - BOSU – Can use foam pad, stair step or box

Lie on your back with your feet planted on top of the Bosu and knees bent. Lift up your buttocks as shown. Hold and then lower yourself slowly and repeat.
Brace the stomach muscles to keep your spine from moving, trying to keep the pelvis level the entire time.

| | _____ Reps _____ Sets _____X Day _____Hold | | _____ Reps _____ Sets _____X Day _____Hold |
|---|---|---|---|
| **7** | **Notes:** | **8** | **Notes:** |

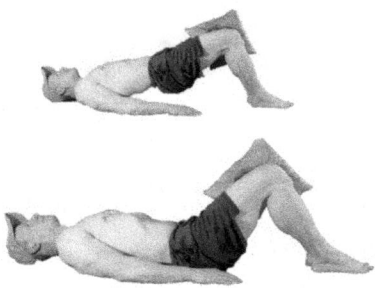

Starting

Position

BRIDGING WITH PILLOW SQUEEZE - Use pillow, ball or rolled towel between knees

Lie on your back and place a pillow, towel roll or ball between your knees and squeeze. Hold this and then tighten your lower abdominals, squeeze your buttocks and raise your buttocks off the floor/bed. Brace the stomach muscles to keep your spine from moving, trying to keep the pelvis level.

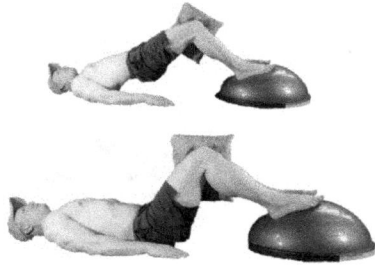

Starting

Position

BRIDGING WITH PILLOW SQUEEZE - BOSU - Can use foam pad, stair step or box

Lie on your back with your feet planted on top of the Bosu and knees bent. Place a pillow, towel roll or ball between your knees and squeeze. Lift up your buttocks as shown. Hold and then lower yourself slowly and repeat. Brace the stomach muscles to keep your spine from moving, trying to keep the pelvis level.

| | _____ Reps _____ Sets _____ X Day _____ Hold |
|---|---|
| **9** | **Notes:** |

Starting Position

BRACE SUPINE MARCHING / BRIDGE LEG UP

Lie on your back with your knees bent, slowly lift up one foot a few inches and then set it back down. Perform on your other leg. Brace the stomach muscles to keep your spine from moving, trying to keep the pelvis level the entire time.
*To increase challenge, go into bridge position as with #5, then continue march – can bring leg higher to advance

| | _____ Reps _____ Sets _____ X Day _____ Hold |
|---|---|
| **10** | **Notes:** |

Starting Position

BRIDGE LEG UP - BOSU - Can use foam pad, stair step or box

Lie on your back with your feet planted on top of the Bosu and knees bent. Slowly lift up one foot a few inches and then set it back down. Next, perform on your other leg. Brace the stomach muscles to keep your spine from moving, trying to keep the pelvis level the entire time. *To increase challenge, go into bridge position as with #6, then continue march – can bring leg higher to advance

| | _____ Reps _____ Sets _____ X Day _____ Hold |
|---|---|
| **11** | **Notes:** |

Starting Position

SINGLE LEG BRIDGE

Lie on your back, raise your buttocks off the floor/bed into a bridge position. Straighten a leg so that only one leg is supporting your body. Then, return that leg back to the ground and change to the other side. Brace the stomach muscles to keep your spine from moving, trying to keep the pelvis level the entire time.

| | _____ Reps _____ Sets _____ X Day _____ Hold |
|---|---|
| **12** | **Notes:** |

Starting Position

BRIDGE SINGLE LEG - BOSU - can use foam pad, stair step or box

Lie on your back with your feet planted on top of the Bosu and knees bent, lift up your buttocks and then straighten one knee in the air. Return that leg back to the ground and change to the other side. Brace the stomach muscles to keep your spine from moving, trying to keep the pelvis level the entire time.

|  | _____ Reps _____ Sets _____X Day _____Hold |  | _____ Reps _____ Sets _____X Day _____Hold |
|---|---|---|---|
| 13 | **Notes:** | 14 | **Notes:** |

Starting Position

**BRIDGING CROSSED LEG**

Lie on your back, cross your leg. Tighten your lower abdomen, squeeze your buttocks and raise your buttocks off the floor/bed. Brace the stomach muscles to keep your spine from moving, trying to keep the pelvis level the entire time.

Starting Position

**BRIDGING CROSSED LEG – BOSU - can use foam pad, stair step or box**

Lie on your back with your feet planted on top of the Bosu cross your leg. Tighten your lower abdomen, squeeze your buttocks and raise your buttocks. Brace the stomach muscles to keep your spine from moving, trying to keep the pelvis level the entire time.

|  | _____ Reps _____ Sets _____X Day _____Hold |  | _____ Reps _____ Sets _____X Day _____Hold |
|---|---|---|---|
| 15 | **Notes:** | 16 | **Notes:** |

Starting Position

**BRIDGING CROSSED LEG - ARMS UP**

Lie on your back, cross your leg and put your hands together as shown. Next, tighten your lower abdomen, squeeze your buttocks and raise your buttocks off the floor/bed. Brace the stomach muscles to keep your spine from moving, trying to keep the pelvis level the entire time.

**BRIDGING CROSSED LEG - ARMS UP - BOSU - can use foam pad, stair step or box**

Lie on your back with your feet planted on top of the Bosu and hands together and leg crossed. Tighten your lower abdomen, squeeze your buttocks and raise your buttocks. Brace the stomach muscles to keep your spine from moving, trying to keep the pelvis level.

| | _____ Reps _____ Sets _____X Day _____Hold | | _____ Reps _____ Sets _____X Day _____Hold |
|---|---|---|---|
| **17** | **Notes:** | **18** | **Notes:** |

Starting Position

**BRIDGE - ELASTIC BAND**

Lie on your back, hold an elastic band down around your waist for resistance. Tighten your lower abdomen, squeeze your buttocks and then raise your buttocks off the floor/bed. Brace the stomach muscles to keep your spine from moving, trying to keep the pelvis level the entire time.

Starting Position

**BRIDGING - ABDUCTION - ELASTIC BAND** – can be done with feet on BOSU, foam, stair step or box

Lie on your back, place an elastic band around your knees and pull your knees apart. Hold this and then tighten your lower abdomen, squeeze your buttocks and raise your buttocks off the floor/bed. Brace the stomach muscles to keep your spine from moving, trying to keep the pelvis level the entire time.

| | _____ Reps _____ Sets _____X Day _____Hold | | _____ Reps _____ Sets _____X Day _____Hold |
|---|---|---|---|
| **19** | **Notes:** | **20** | **Notes:** |

Starting Position

**FLOOR BRIDGE - EXERCISE BALL**

Lie on the floor, place an exercise ball under your lower legs and then raise up your buttocks. Hold and repeat. Brace the stomach muscles to keep your spine from moving, trying to keep the pelvis level the entire time.

Starting Position

**FLOOR BRIDGE ALTERNATE LEG LIFT - EXERCISE BALL**

Lie on the floor, place an exercise ball under your lower legs and then raise up your buttocks. While holding this position raise up a leg off the ball towards the ceiling then lower back to the ball and alternate to lift the other leg. Brace the stomach muscles to keep your spine from moving, trying to keep the pelvis level.

| _____ Reps _____ Sets _____X Day _____Hold | | _____ Reps _____ Sets _____X Day _____Hold |
|---|---|---|
| **21** | **Notes:** | **22** | **Notes:** |

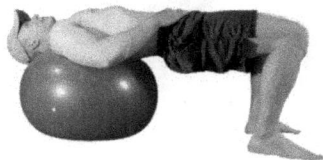

**BRIDGE UPPER BACK - EXERCISE BALL**

Start in a seated position on the ball and slowly walk your feet forward so that the ball is on your upper back. Keep your buttocks and pelvis up off the ball and straight with your thighs. Brace the stomach muscles to keep your spine from moving, trying to keep the pelvis level the entire time.
*To increase the challenge, you can do a supine march or perform some arm exercises, such as Fly's or Chest Presses (*See Upper Extremity exercises*)

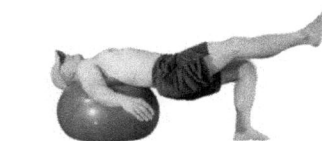

Starting Position

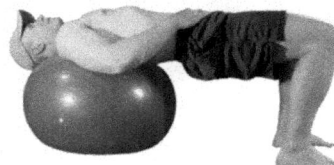

**BRIDGE UPPER BACK - SINGLE LEG - EXERCISE BALL**

Start in a seated position on the ball and slowly walk your feet forward so that the ball is on your upper back. Keep your buttocks and pelvis up off the ball and straight with your thighs. Raise up one leg so that you straighten your knee in the air. Return it back to the floor and then switch to raise up the other side. Brace the stomach muscles to keep your spine from moving, trying to keep the pelvis level the entire time.

## Quadruped

| _____ Reps _____ Sets _____X Day _____Hold | | _____ Reps _____ Sets _____X Day _____Hold |
|---|---|---|
| **23** | **Notes:** | **24** | **Notes:** |

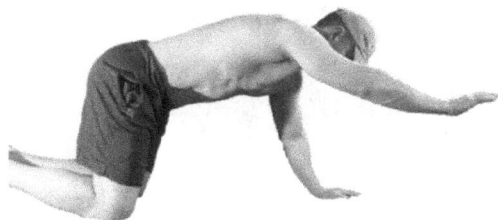

**QUADRUPED ALTERNATE ARM**

While in a crawling position, slowly raise up an arm out in front of you.

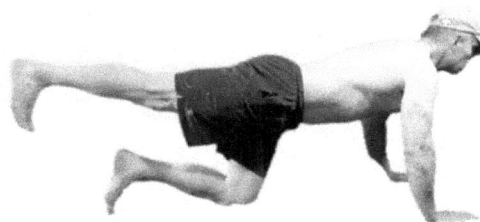

**QUADRUPED ALTERNATE LEG**

While in a crawling position, slowly draw your leg back behind you as you straighten your knee. Either repeat on same side or alternate.

| \_\_\_\_\_ Reps \_\_\_\_\_ Sets \_\_\_\_\_X Day \_\_\_\_\_Hold |
| --- |

**25** | **Notes:**

QUADRUPED ALTERNATE ARM AND LEG

While in a crawling position, brace at your abdominals and then slowly lift a leg and opposite arm upwards. Maintain a level and stable pelvis and spine the entire time. Either repeat on same side or alternate.

| \_\_\_\_\_ Reps \_\_\_\_\_ Sets \_\_\_\_\_X Day \_\_\_\_\_Hold |
| --- |

**26** | **Notes:**

Touch your elbow to your opposite knee

Starting Position

BIRD DOG ELBOW TOUCHES

While in a crawling position, slowly lift your leg and opposite arm upwards. When returning your arm and leg down, do not touch the floor but instead touch your elbow to your opposite knee and lift and straighten them again. Then set them down on the floor. Either repeat on same side or alternate.

| \_\_\_\_\_ Reps \_\_\_\_\_ Sets \_\_\_\_\_X Day \_\_\_\_\_Hold |
| --- |

**27** | **Notes:**

PRONE BALL

Lie face down over a ball, support your self with your feet and hands.

| \_\_\_\_\_ Reps \_\_\_\_\_ Sets \_\_\_\_\_X Day \_\_\_\_\_Hold |
| --- |

**28** | **Notes:**

PRONE BALL - ALTERNATE ARM

Lie face down over a ball, support your self with your feet and hands. Next, slowly raise up one arm. Return arm back to floor and then raise up the other arm. Keep alternating arms.

| _____ Reps _____ Sets _____X Day _____Hold | _____ Reps _____ Sets _____X Day _____Hold |
|---|---|
| **29** Notes: | **30** Notes: |

PRONE BALL - ALTERNATE LEG

Lie face down over a ball, support yourself with your arms and legs. Next slowly raise up a leg. Return leg back to floor and then raise up the other leg.

PRONE BALL - ALTERNATE ARM AND LEG

Lie face down over a ball, support yourself with your feet and hands. Next, slowly raise up one arm and opposite leg. Return arm and leg back to floor and then raise up the opposite arm/leg.

## Plank

| _____ Reps _____ Sets _____X Day _____Hold | _____ Reps _____ Sets _____X Day _____Hold |
|---|---|
| **31** Notes: | **32** Notes: |

MODIFIED PLANK

Lie face down, lift your body up on your elbows and toes. Try and maintain a straight spine the entire time. Do not allow your low back sag downward.

Starting Position

MODIFIED PLANK - ALTERNATE LEG

Lie face down, lift your body up on your elbows and toes. Next, lift one leg off the ground and then set it back down. Then repeat on the other leg. Try and maintain a straight spine the entire time.

_____ Reps _____ Sets _____X Day _____Hold

**33** | Notes:

FULL PLANK

Lie face down, lift your body up on your elbows and toes. Straighten your arms in full elbow extension and hold in full plank position. Do not let your back arch down. Try and maintain a straight spine the entire time.

_____ Reps _____ Sets _____X Day _____Hold

**34** | Notes:

PLANK - ALTERNATE ARMS

Hold a plank position as previous (#33). Raise one arm out in front of you as shown. Return to the starting position and then raise your other arm out in front of you and repeat.
Try and maintain a straight spine the entire time.

_____ Reps _____ Sets _____X Day _____Hold

**35** | Notes:

PLANK - ALTERNATE LEGS

Hold a plank position as previous (#33). Raise one leg off the floor as shown. Return to the starting position and then raise your other leg and repeat. Try and maintain a straight spine the entire time.

_____ Reps _____ Sets _____X Day _____Hold

**36** | Notes:

PLANK - EXERCISE BALL

While kneeling on the floor with an exercise ball in front of you, place your elbows and hands on the ball and lift your body up. Try and maintain a straight spine. Do not allow your hips or pelvis on either side to drop.

## Back Extension

| _____ Reps _____ Sets _____X Day _____Hold | | _____ Reps _____ Sets _____X Day _____Hold |
|---|---|---|
| **37** Notes: | | **38** Notes: |

### PRONE ON ELBOWS

Lie face down, slowly press up and prop yourself up on your elbows.

### PRESS UPS

Lie face down, slowly press up and arch your back using your arms.

| _____ Reps _____ Sets _____X Day _____Hold | | _____ Reps _____ Sets _____X Day _____Hold |
|---|---|---|
| **39** Notes: | | **40** Notes: |

### SKYDIVER

Lie face down with arms by your side. Next, lift your upper body, lower legs, thighs, and arms off the ground at the same time as shown. You can place a pillow under your stomach/hips for comfort.

### PRONE SUPERMAN - BOSU

Lie face down over the Bosu. Slowly raise your arms and legs upward off the ground. Then lower slowly back to the ground.

|  | _____ Reps _____ Sets _____X Day _____Hold |
|---|---|
| **41** | **Notes:** |

Starting

Position

**TRUNK EXTENSION - BOSU**

Lie face down with your upper body on a Bosu and slowly raise your head and chest upwards as shown.
Your arms can be behind your back or alongside your body.

|  | _____ Reps _____ Sets _____X Day _____Hold |
|---|---|
| **42** | **Notes:** |

Starting

Position

**TRUNK EXTENSION - HANDS BEHIND HEAD - BOSU**

Lie face down with your upper body on a Bosu. Touch the back of your head with both hands and slowly raise your head and chest upwards.

|  | _____ Reps _____ Sets _____X Day _____Hold |
|---|---|
| **43** | **Notes:** |

Starting

Position

**TRUNK EXTENSION - HANDS CROSSED IN FRONT - BOSU**

While lying face down with your upper body on a Bosu, slowly raise your head and chest upwards.
Keep your arms crossed on your chest as you perform.

|  | _____ Reps _____ Sets _____X Day _____Hold |
|---|---|
| **44** | **Notes:** |

**SUPERMAN - ARMS BACK- EXERCISE BALL**

Start in a kneeling position with an exercise ball in front of you. Roll forward so that you are face down on the ball with your feet on the ground and your stomach on the ball. Hold up your head and chest so that a straight line exists between your feet and head. Also bring your arms back along side of your body and hold this position.

| | _____ Reps _____ Sets _____ X Day _____ Hold | | | _____ Reps _____ Sets _____ X Day _____ Hold |
|---|---|---|---|---|
| 45 | Notes: | | 46 | Notes: |

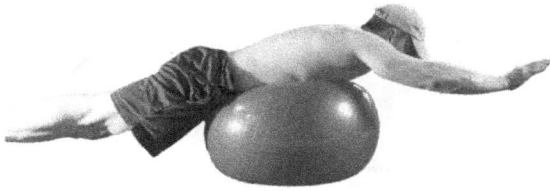

**SUPERMAN – BOTH ARMS IN FRONT - EXERCISE BALL**

Start in a kneeling position with an exercise ball in front of you. Next, roll forward so that you are face down on the ball with your feet on the ground and your stomach on the ball. Hold up your head and chest so that a straight line exists between your feet and head. Also bring your arms up and forward out in front of you and hold this position.

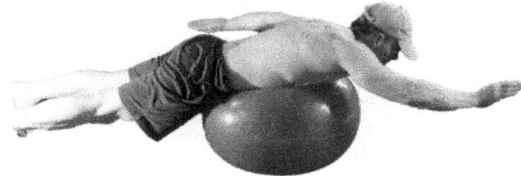

**SUPERMAN – ONE ARM FORWARD / ONE ARM BACK - EXERCISE BALL**

Start in a kneeling position with an exercise ball in front of you. Next, roll forward so that you are face down on the ball with your feet on the ground and your stomach on the ball. Hold up your head and chest so that a straight line exists between your feet and head. Raise one arm up and out in front of you as you bring the other arm back and along side your body as in a swimming motion.

## Lateral Plank

| | _____ Reps _____ Sets _____ X Day _____ Hold | | | _____ Reps _____ Sets _____ X Day _____ Hold |
|---|---|---|---|---|
| 47 | Notes: | | 48 | Notes: |

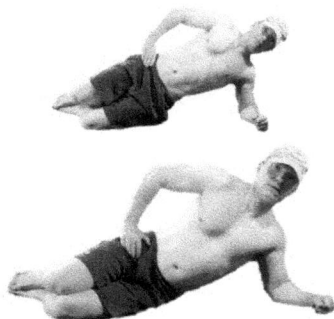

Starting Position

**LATERAL PLANK MODIFIED**

Lie on your side with your knees bent, lift your body up on your elbow and knees. Try and maintain a straight spine.

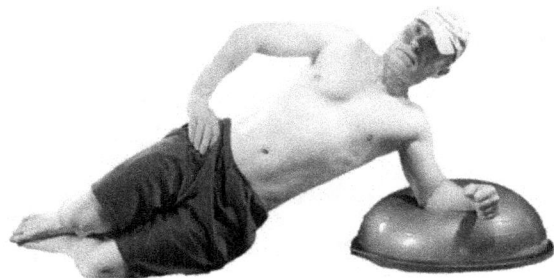

**LATERAL PLANK MODIFIED- BOSU- can be anything unstable**

Lie on your side with your knees bent and your elbow on the Bosu, lift your body up on your elbow and knees. Try and maintain a straight spine.

| _____ Reps _____ Sets _____ X Day _____ Hold | | _____ Reps _____ Sets _____ X Day _____ Hold | |
|---|---|---|---|
| **49** | **Notes:** | **50** | **Notes:** |

**LATERAL PLANK - 1 KNEE 1 FOOT**

Lie on your side with bottom knee bent and top knee straight. Lift your body up on your elbow and knee on one side and foot on the other side. Try and maintain a straight spine.

**LATERAL PLANK - 1 KNEE 1 FOOT – BOSU- Can be anything unstable**

Lie on your side with elbow on Bosu with bottom knee bent and the top knee straight. Lift your body up on your elbow and knee on one side and foot on the other side. Try and maintain a straight spine.

| _____ Reps _____ Sets _____ X Day _____ Hold | | _____ Reps _____ Sets _____ X Day _____ Hold | |
|---|---|---|---|
| **51** | **Notes:** | **52** | **Notes:** |

Starting Position

**LATERAL PLANK**

Lie on your side with both legs straight and lift your body up on your elbow and feet. Try and maintain a straight spine.

**LATERAL PLANK - BOSU - Can be anything unstable**

Lie on your side with your elbow on the Bosu and both legs straight. Lift your body up on your elbow and feet. Try and maintain a straight spine.

## Backward Lean

| | | | |
|---|---|---|---|
| _____ Reps _____ Sets _____ X Day _____ Hold | | | |

**53** | **Notes:**

Starting
Position

LEAN BACK

Start in an upright seated position with knees bent.  Hold onto thighs and lean back keeping spine as straight as possible.

| | | | |
|---|---|---|---|
| _____ Reps _____ Sets _____ X Day _____ Hold | | | |

**54** | **Notes:**

Starting
Position

LEAN BACK - BOSU

Start in an upright seated position on Bosu with knees bent.  Hold onto thighs or Bosu and lean back keeping spine as straight as possible.

| | | | |
|---|---|---|---|
| _____ Reps _____ Sets _____ X Day _____ Hold | | | |

**55** | **Notes:**

Starting
Position

LEAN BACK WITH ARMS OUT

Start in an upright seated position with knees bent.  Hold arms straight out or overhead, brace core and lean back keeping spine as straight as possible

| | | | |
|---|---|---|---|
| _____ Reps _____ Sets _____ X Day _____ Hold | | | |

**56** | **Notes:**

Starting
Position

LEAN BACK WITH ARMS OUT  - BOSU

Start in an upright seated position on  Bosu with knees bent.  Hold arms straight out or overhead, brace core and lean back keeping spine as straight as possible.

| | Reps | Sets | X Day | Hold |
|---|---|---|---|---|

**57**  Notes:

Starting

Position

LEAN BACK WITH TWIST

Start in an upright seated position with knees bent.  Hold arms straight out, brace core and lean back keeping spine as straight as possible.  Rotate trunk/arms to one side and then repeat to the other side.

| | Reps | Sets | X Day | Hold |
|---|---|---|---|---|

**58**  Notes:

Starting

Position

LEAN BACK WITH TWIST – BOSU

Start in an upright seated position on  Bosu with knees bent.  Hold arms straight out, brace core and lean back keeping spine as straight as possible.  Rotate trunk/arms to one side - repeat to the other side

| | Reps | Sets | X Day | Hold |
|---|---|---|---|---|

**59**  Notes:

CRUNCHY FROG

Sit on floor or edge of couch/bench.  Lean back and with arms wide apart and legs straight.  Next, bring knees towards chest and arms forward and return to starting position.

| | Reps | Sets | X Day | Hold |
|---|---|---|---|---|

**60**  Notes:

SEATED BIKE - FORWARD AND BACKWARDS

Sit on floor and lean back.  With arms on floor or off ground, peddle feet forward for 15-30 repetitions, rest and then reverse.  *Progress by moving hands forward near hips or remove arm support*

# Abdominal Crunch Variations

| | _____ Reps _____ Sets _____ X Day _____ Hold |
|---|---|
| **61** | **Notes:** |

Starting Position

**CRUNCH – ARMS OUT**

Lie on your back with your arms outstretched forward, brace core and curl up lifting your shoulder blades off the ground. Exhale as you come up and squeeze/tighten your abdominal muscles.

| | _____ Reps _____ Sets _____ X Day _____ Hold |
|---|---|
| **62** | **Notes:** |

Starting Position

**CRUNCH – ARMS OUT - BOSU**

Lie on your back on Bosu with your arms outstretched forward, brace core and curl up lifting your shoulder blades off the ground. Exhale as you come up and squeeze/tighten your abdominal muscles.

| | _____ Reps _____ Sets _____ X Day _____ Hold |
|---|---|
| **63** | **Notes:** |

Starting Position

**CRUNCH – ARMS IN BACK OF HEAD**

Lie on your back with your arms behind your head, brace core and curl up lifting your shoulder blades off the ground. Exhale as you come up and squeeze/tighten your abdominal muscles. Do not pull on your neck/head.

| | _____ Reps _____ Sets _____ X Day _____ Hold |
|---|---|
| **64** | **Notes:** |

**CRUNCH – ARMS IN BACK OF HEAD - BOSU**

Lie on your back on Bosu with your arms behind your head, brace core and curl up lifting your shoulder blades off the ground. Exhale as you come up and squeeze/tighten your abdominal muscles. Do not pull on your neck/head.

| | |
|---|---|
| _____ Reps _____ Sets _____ X Day _____ Hold | _____ Reps _____ Sets _____ X Day _____ Hold |
| **65** Notes: | **66** Notes: |

**OBLIQUE CRUNCH**

Lie on your back with one or both hands in back of head. Brace core and curl up targeting elbow to opposite knee as shown. Keep shoulders off floor. Exhale as you come up and squeeze/tighten your abdominal muscles. Do not pull on your neck/head.

**OBLIQUE CRUNCH - BOSU**

Lie back on Bosu with one or both hands in back of head. Brace core and curl up targeting elbow to opposite knee as shown. Keep shoulders off Bosu. Exhale as you come up and squeeze/tighten your abdominal muscles. Do not pull on your neck/head.

| | |
|---|---|
| _____ Reps _____ Sets _____ X Day _____ Hold | _____ Reps _____ Sets _____ X Day _____ Hold |
| **67** Notes: | **68** Notes: |

**90 DEGREE CRUNCH**

Lie on your back with legs straight in air. Reach your hands towards toes, crunching shoulders off ground. Exhale as you come up and squeeze/tighten your abdominal muscles.

**BALL CRUNCH – Can put legs on seat of chair**

Lie on back with legs up on ball so knees and hips are at ~ 90 degrees. Cross hands over chest or behind head. Brace core and curl up lifting your shoulder blades off the ground. Exhale as you come up and squeeze/tighten your abdominal muscles. Do not pull on your neck/head.

| | _____ Reps _____ Sets _____ X Day _____ Hold | | _____ Reps _____ Sets _____ X Day _____ Hold |
|---|---|---|---|
| **69** | **Notes:** | **70** | **Notes:** |

Starting

Position

CURL UPS – ARMS ON LEGS - EXERCISE BALL

While sitting on an exercise ball, roll forward so that your back lies against the ball. Put hands on thighs/legs. Brace core and curl up lifting your shoulder blades off the ball. Exhale as you come up and squeeze/tighten your abdominal muscles.

CURL UPS- ARMS CROSSED IN FRONT - EXERCISE BALL

While sitting on an exercise ball, roll forward so that your back lies against the ball. Cross hands over your chest. Brace core and curl up lifting your shoulder blades off the ball. Exhale as you come up and squeeze/tighten your abdominal muscles.

| | _____ Reps _____ Sets _____ X Day _____ Hold | | _____ Reps _____ Sets _____ X Day _____ Hold |
|---|---|---|---|
| **71** | **Notes:** | **72** | **Notes:** |

Starting   Position

CURL UPS – ARMS BEHIND HEAD - EXERCISE BALL

While sitting on an exercise ball, roll forward so that your back lies against the ball. Place your hands behind your head. Brace core and curl up lifting your shoulder blades off the ball. Exhale as you come up and squeeze/tighten your abdominal muscles. Do not pull on your neck/head.

SUPINE CRUNCH TOUCH - EXERCISE BALL

Lie on the floor with your knees bend and holding a ball over your head. Bring both your knees and ball towards each other above your chest and touch your knees to the ball. Slowly return both to original positions and repeat.

_____ Reps _____ Sets _____X Day _____Hold

**73** **Notes:**

_____ Reps _____ Sets _____X Day _____Hold

**74** **Notes:**

LOWER ABDOMINAL CRUNCH – WITH or WITHOUT BALL

Sit on a solid surface with or without a ball/pillow between your knees. Maintaining a straight spine, contract your lower abdominals. Lift both knees up. Hold and control movement back to starting position. Repeat. Can be done holding onto surface for added stability with or without ball (3rd picture)

HIGH MARCH CRUNCH

Lift knee towards chest keeping hips forward in a high march position. Continue to alternate sides while standing in place. Exhale as you come up and squeeze/tighten your abdominal muscles.

_____ Reps _____ Sets _____X Day _____Hold

**75** **Notes:**

_____ Reps _____ Sets _____X Day _____Hold

**76** **Notes:**

Starting Position

STANDING SIDE CRUNCH

Standing with hip rotated out bring knee up towards same side elbow squeezing your obliques. Continue alternating sides while standing in place. Exhale as you come up and squeeze/tighten muscles.

Starting Position

STANDING BIKE CRUNCH

Lift knee to chest and rotate pulling opposite elbow towards knee. Continue to alternate sides while standing in place. Exhale as you come up and squeeze/tighten muscles.

# Strengthening

## Anaerobic - without oxygen:  Single repetition with maximum resistance

Lifting lighter weights with a high number of repetitions will result in 'toning', whereas lifting heavier weights with a lower number of repetitions will result in 'bulking up'.

| | |
|---|---|
| **Benefits of strengthening** | • Increases muscle fiber size and contractile strength<br>• Increases tendon and ligament strength<br>• Increases bone strength / bone mineral density<br>• Improves hormonal balances-decreased cortisol<br>• Increases Peripheral (PNS) and Central (CNS) Nervous System communication/proprioception<br>• Improves function for ADL's (Activities of Daily Living) |
| **Range of Motion (ROM)** | Refers to the distance and direction a joint can move between the flexed position and the extended position (stretching from flexion to extension for physiological gain).  It is important to be able to complete full ROM before adding resistance. ***Before strengthening (adding resistance), make sure you can go through full ROM*** unless being followed by an MD or physical/occupational therapist or other professional. |
| **Forms of strengthening exercise** | • **Isometric** – Muscles contract with no motion at the joint or change in length of the muscle.  The exercises usually consist of maximal effort against an object that does not move, like a wall.<br>• **Isotonic** – Muscles contract with motion at the joint; muscles either lengthen or shorten (*see **concentric/eccentric** below*).  Tension is not constant through the range of motion. (During a bicep curl, holding a 5 lb weight, the contraction is not constant during the entire movement).  Most common form of isotonic exercises use free weights with either dumbbells or a barbell.<br>• **Concentric** – Muscle shortens, positive phase of lift.  Bending the elbow in a bicep curl<br>• **Eccentric** – Muscle lengthens, negative phase of lift or lowering. Straightening the elbow in a bicep curl.<br>• **Isokinetic** – Muscles contract with motion at the joint; muscles either lengthen or shorten.  Machines or equipment control the speed of the movement, so tension is constant providing the maximum amount of resistance throughout the entire movement. |
| **Repetition (Reps)** | Single cycle of lifting and lowering a weight in a controlled manner, moving through the form of the exercise.  Example:  12 Bicep curls per set. |
| **Set** | Several repetitions performed one after another with no break between.  There can be a number of reps per set and sets per exercise depending on the goal of the individual. Example:  12 reps x3 sets |
| **Rep Maximum (RM)** | The number of repetitions one can perform at a certain weight is called the Rep Maximum (RM). For example, if one could perform 10 repetitions with a 75 lbs dumbbell, then their RM for that weight would be 10RM.<br>1RM is the maximum weight that someone can lift in a given exercise - i.e. a weight that they can only lift once. (*Wikipedia*) (*See Bulk Up or Tone Up Below*) |
| **Bulk up or Tone up** | Do you want to 'bulk up' or 'tone up'?  Although much of this depends on genetics and your ratio of slow and fast twitch fibers, discussed in the *Endurance* section, it is good to know what your goals are before starting.  The average person should be able to perform at about 75% of their maximum resistance for 10 repetitions.  If you can do ONE bicep curl with a 20-pound dumbbell/weight, then you should be able to do 10 with a 15 lbs. weight. (See *Set*)  20 lbs. x 75% = 15 lbs.  Once you get into a routine, it will be easy for you to know when to increase the weight. |

| | |
|---|---|
| **General rule of thumb** | • Work from the Ground up<br>• Order: Isometric > ROM > Eccentric > Concentric<br>• Use assistance before resistance – Start without weight to complete range of motion and then add weight with proper form. *(See ROM above)*<br>• Add weight: 8-12 reps x 2-3 sets of each exercise at 75% of one repetition maximum (one-rep max).<br>• Once you reach 12 easily, you can then recheck your one-rep max. If it has increased, then increase your weight as above.<br>• If you are looking to 'bulk up', perform low repetitions at a higher weight – up to 85-90% of the one-rep maximum. 5-8 reps x 2-3 sets. With increased weight, there is a higher risk of injury.<br>• If you are looking to 'tone up', perform high repetitions with 65-75% of the one-rep max. 12-20 reps x 2-3 sets.<br>• Do NOT exercise the same muscle group every day. The muscles need about 48-72 hours to repair. This includes the abdomen.<br>**Muscle strengthening, if you are lifting weights, alternate upper and lower body with isolated abdomen exercises every other day as well. For those working out several days a week, find a schedule that works for you, but give each muscle group 48-72 hours to recover.<br>• Cardiac/aerobic conditioning can be done daily.<br>• Breathe!! Always exhale on the exertion. For example, when you are doing a crunch, exhale as you flexing the abs or 'curling'. Do not hold your breath.<br>• Engage your core. Don't forget what you learned under core and balance. |

## Duration, Frequency, Intensity and Movement Patterns

| | |
|---|---|
| **Intensity:**<br><br>How *much* mental and physical *effort* it takes to sustain an activity. | This can be done using the target heart rate range THR (optimum exercise intensity levels through beats per minute, talk test or rate of perceived exertion. |
| **Duration:**<br><br>How *long* the training lasts. | The higher the intensity, the shorter the duration. The American College of Sports Medicine guidelines recommend all healthy adults aged 18–65 yr should participate in moderate intensity aerobic physical activity for a minimum of 30 min on five days per week, or vigorous intensity aerobic activity for a minimum of 20 min on three days per week. |
| **Frequency:**<br><br>How *often* the training occurs. | Strength training should be performed every other day or 2-3 days a week. It is important to give each muscle group 48-72 hours to recover. Alternate upper and lower body with isolated abdomen/core exercises every other day. For those working out several days a week, find a schedule that works for you as long as you give each muscle group 48 hours of recovery time. |
| **Movement Patterns and Examples**<br><br>Basic movements that help to increase overall body strengthening | • Bend and Lift: Squats, Dead Lifts and Leg presses<br>  o Picking up item off floor<br>• Single Leg: Step ups, Single leg stance, Lunges<br>  o Walking up steps<br>• Push: Shoulder press, Bench press, Push up<br>  o Pushing Shopping cart or Lawn mower<br>• Pull: Lat pull downs, Seated rows<br>  o Vacuuming, Raking<br>• Rotational<br>  o Shoveling snow |

| EXERCISE<br><br>Lower Extremity - Lying & Seated<br>Strengthening and Range of Motion | EXERCISE NUMBER | NOTES |
|---|---|---|
| INVERSION – SEATED - ELASTIC BAND | 1 | |
| INVERSION – SEATED - ELASTIC BAND - 2 | 2 | |
| EVERSION – SEATED - ELASTIC BAND | 3 | |
| EVERSION – SEATED - ELASTIC BAND - 2 | 4 | |
| ANKLE PUMPS - SEATED | 5 | |
| ANKLE PUMPS – SUPINE or FEET UP ON STOOL | 6 | |
| DORSIFLEXION – SEATED - ELASTIC BAND | 7 | |
| DORSIFLEXION – SEATED - ELASTIC BAND - 2 | 8 | |
| PLANTARFLEXION - STRAP | 9 | |
| PLANTARFLEXION - SEATED – ELASTIC BAND | 10 | |
| HEEL SLIDES - SUPINE | 11 | |
| HEEL SLIDES - RESISTED EXTENSION – ELASTIC BAND | 12 | |
| QUAD SET –ISOMETRIC | 13 | |
| QUAD SET WITH TOWEL UNDER HEEL - ISOMETRIC | 14 | |
| SHORT ARC QUAD (SAQ) – SELF ASSISTED | 15 | |
| SHORT ARC QUAD - (SAQ) | 16 | |
| KNEE EXTENSION - SELF ASSISTED | 17 | |
| PARTIAL ARC QUAD - LOW SEAT | 18 | |
| LONG ARC QUAD (LAQ) – LOW SEAT (90 deg) | 19 | |
| LONG ARC QUAD (LAQ) – LOW SEAT - ANKLE WEIGHTS | 20 | |
| LONG ARC QUAD (LAQ) - HIGH SEAT | 21 | |
| LONG ARC QUAD (LAQ) - HIGH SEAT - ANKLE WEIGHTS | 22 | |
| LONG ARC QUAD - ELASTIC BAND – HAND HELD | 23 | |
| LONG ARC QUAD - ELASTIC BAND | 24 | |

**Lower Extremity Strengthening**

| EXERCISE<br>Lower Extremity - Lying & Seated<br>Strengthening and Range of Motion | EXERCISE NUMBER | NOTES |
|---|---|---|
| HAMSTRING CURLS - PRONE - ASSISTED | 25 | |
| HAMSTRING CURLS - PRONE | 26 | |
| HAMSTRING CURLS - - PRONE - WEIGHTS | 27 | |
| HAMSTRING CURLS – PRONE - ELASTIC BAND | 28 | |
| HAMSTRING CURLS – ELASTIC BAND | 29 | |
| HAMSTRING CURLS – ELASTIC BAND - 2 | 30 | |
| HAMSTRING CURLS ON BALL | 31 | |
| HAMSTRING CURLS - SINGLE LEG - EXERCISE BALL | 32 | |
| HIP FLEXION ISOMETRIC | 33 | |
| HIP FLEXION ISOMETRIC BILATERAL | 34 | |
| HIP FLEXION – ISOMETRIC | 35 | |
| STRAIGHT LEG RAISE (SLR) | 36 | |
| STRAIGHT LEG RAISE (SLR) – ANKLE WEIGHTS | 37 | |
| STRAIGHT LEG RAISE (SLR) - ELASTIC BAND | 38 | |
| SEATED MARCHING | 39 | |
| SEATED MARCHING - ELASTIC BAND | 40 | |
| HIP EXTENSION - PRONE | 41 | |
| HIP EXTENSION – PRONE – ANKLE WEIGHTS | 42 | |
| HIP EXTENSION – PRONE – ELASTIC BAND | 43 | |
| HIP EXTENSION – QUADRUPED | 44 | |
| HIP ABDUCTION - SUPINE | 45 | |
| HIP ABDUCTION - SUPINE – ANKLE WEIGHTS | 46 | |
| HIP ABDUCTION – SUPINE - ELASTIC BAND | 47 | |
| HIP ABDUCTION / CLAMS– SUPINE - ELASTIC BAND | 48 | |
| MODIFIED HIP ABDUCTION – SIDELYING | 49 | |

| EXERCISE<br><br>Lower Extremity - Lying & Seated<br>Strengthening and Range of Motion | EXERCISE<br>NUMBER | NOTES |
|---|---|---|
| HIP ABDUCTION – SIDELYING | 50 | |
| HIP ABDUCTION – SIDELYING - WEIGHTS | 51 | |
| HIP ABDUCTION – SIDELYING - ELASTIC BAND | 52 | |
| CLAM SHELLS | 53 | |
| SIDELYING CLAM - ELASTIC BAND | 54 | |
| HIP ABDUCTION - FIRE HYDRANT - QUADRUPED | 55 | |
| HIP ABDUCTION - FIRE HYDRANT – QUADRUPED - ELASTIC BAND | 56 | |
| HIP ABDUCTION - SEATED - STRAIGHT LEG | 57 | |
| HIP ABDUCTION - SEATED - STRAIGHT LEG – ANKLE WEIGHT | 58 | |
| HIP ABDUCTION - SINGLE- SEATED | 59 | |
| HIP ABDUCTION - SINGLE- SEATED – ELASTIC BAND | 60 | |
| HIP ABDUCTION - BILATERAL- SEATED | 61 | |
| HIP ABDUCTION - BILATERAL- SEATED - ELASTIC BAND | 62 | |
| HIP ADDUCTION SQUEEZE – SUPINE – KNEES BENT | 63 | |
| HIP ADDUCTION SQUEEZE – SUPINE – LEGS STRAIGHT | 64 | |
| HIP ADDUCTION - SIDELYING | 65 | |
| INTERNAL ROTATION - HEEL SQUEEZE - ISOMETRIC | 67 | |
| HIP INTERNAL ROTATION - SUPINE | 68 | |
| REVERSE CLAMS - SIDELYING | 69 | |
| REVERSE CLAMS - SIDELYING - ELASTIC BAND | 70 | |
| HIP INTERNAL ROTATION - SEATED | 71 | |
| HIP INTERNAL ROTATION - ELASTIC BAND | 72 | |
| HIP EXTERNAL ROTATION - SUPINE | 73 | |

| EXERCISE<br><br>Lower Extremity - Lying & Seated<br>Strengthening and Range of Motion | EXERCISE NUMBER | NOTES |
|---|---|---|
| HIP EXTERNAL ROTATION - ELASTIC BAND | 74 | |
| HIP ROTATIONS – BILATERAL - SIDELYING | 75 | |
| HIP ROTATION - SEATED - BALL and ELASTIC BAND | 76 | |
| PRESS – BILATERAL – ELASTIC BAND | 77 | |
| PRESS – SINGLE LEG – ELASTIC BAND | 78 | |
| HIP HIKE - STANDING | 79 | |
| HIP HIKE – KNEELING | 80 | |
| GLUTE SETS - PRONE | 81 | |
| GLUTE SET - SUPINE | 82 | |
| GLUTE SQUEEZE - SITTING | 83 | |
| PT (MAX/MEDIUS) | 84 | |

# LOWER EXTREMITY - Range Of Motion > Isometric > Strength
## *Lying and Seated*

### Inversion (IV) / Eversion (EV)

| | _____ Reps _____ Sets _____ X Day _____ Hold |
|---|---|
| **1** | **Notes:** |

| | _____ Reps _____ Sets _____ X Day _____ Hold |
|---|---|
| **2** | **Notes:** |

**INVERSION – SEATED - ELASTIC BAND**

In a seated position, cross your legs and using an elastic band attached to your foot, hook it under your opposite foot and up to your hand.   Draw the resisted foot inward. Keep your heel in contact with the floor the entire time.

**INVERSION – SEATED - ELASTIC BAND - 2**

In a seated position, use an elastic band secured to a steady object and the other end attached to your foot. Draw the resisted foot inward. Keep your heel in contact with the floor the entire time.

| | _____ Reps _____ Sets _____ X Day _____ Hold |
|---|---|
| **3** | **Notes:** |

| | _____ Reps _____ Sets _____ X Day _____ Hold |
|---|---|
| **4** | **Notes:** |

**EVERSION – SEATED - ELASTIC BAND**

In a seated position, use an elastic band attached to your foot, hook it under your opposite foot and up to your hand. Draw the resisted foot outward. Keep your heel in contact with the floor the entire time.

**EVERSION – SEATED - ELASTIC BAND - 2**

In a seated position, use an elastic band secured to a steady object and the other end attached to your foot. Draw the resisted foot outward. Keep your heel in contact with the floor the entire time.

# Dorsiflexion (DF) / Plantarflexion (PF)

| | _____ Reps _____ Sets _____ X Day _____ Hold |
|---|---|
| **5** | Notes: |

ANKLE PUMPS - SEATED

In a seated position keeping feet on the floor, first go up on toes (toes pointed towards the ground – PF). Then point toes up keeping heels on the ground (DF). Alternate back and forth in a pumping motion.

| | _____ Reps _____ Sets _____ X Day _____ Hold |
|---|---|
| **6** | Notes: |

ANKLE PUMPS – SUPINE or FEET UP ON STOOL

Lying or with feet up on stool first point the toes forward (PF) and then back up with toes facing the ceiling. Alternate back and forth in a pumping motion.

| | _____ Reps _____ Sets _____ X Day _____ Hold |
|---|---|
| **7** | Notes: |

DORSIFLEXION – SEATED - ELASTIC BAND

In a seated position, use an elastic band attached to your target foot, hook it under your opposite foot and up to your hand. Draw the band upwards with the resisted foot as shown. Keep your heel in contact with the floor the entire time.

| | _____ Reps _____ Sets _____ X Day _____ Hold |
|---|---|
| **8** | Notes: |

DORSIFLEXION – SEATED - ELASTIC BAND - 2

In a seated position, use an elastic band secured to a steady object and the other end attached to your foot. Draw the resisted foot upward. Keep your heel in contact with the floor the entire time.

| _____ Reps _____ Sets _____X Day _____Hold | | _____ Reps _____ Sets _____X Day _____Hold |
|---|---|---|
| **9** | **Notes:** | **10** | **Notes:** |

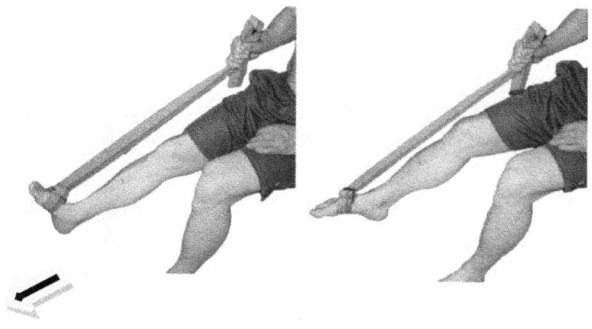

**PLANTARFLEXION - STRAP**

In a seated position, attach one loop of the strap to your foot and hold the other end. Move your foot forward and back at the ankle as shown. Keep your heel in contact with the floor the entire time.

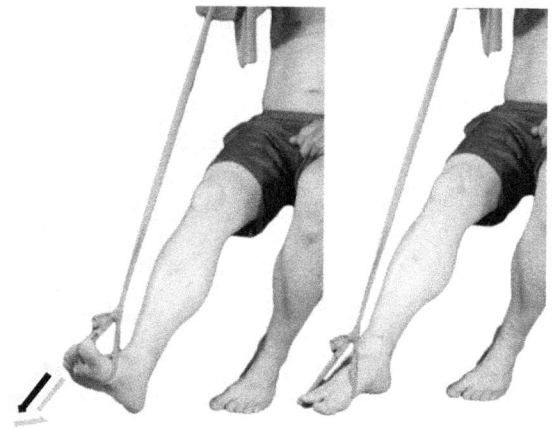

**PLANTARFLEXION - SEATED – ELASTIC BAND**

In a seated position, hold an elastic band and attach the other end to your foot. Press your foot downward towards the floor. Keep your heel in contact with the floor the entire time.

## Heel Slides

| _____ Reps _____ Sets _____X Day _____Hold | | _____ Reps _____ Sets _____X Day _____Hold |
|---|---|---|
| **11** | **Notes:** | **12** | **Notes:** |

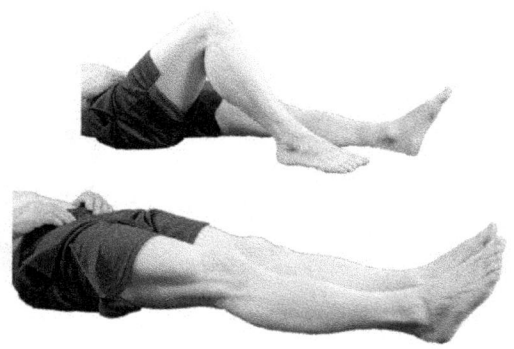

**HEEL SLIDES - SUPINE**

Lie on your back with knees straight and slide the target heel towards your buttock as you bend your knee. Hold a gentle stretch in this position and then return to original position.

Starting Position

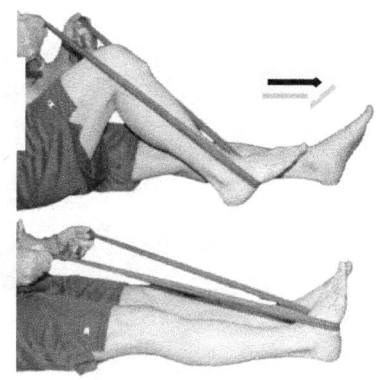

**HEEL SLIDES - RESISTED EXTENSION – ELASTIC BAND**

Long sit with band around bottom of target foot. Slide the target heel towards your buttock as you bend your knee. Push your foot to straighten knee against resistance to the original position.

# Quadriceps (QUAD) / Knee Extension

| | _____ Reps _____ Sets _____X Day _____Hold | | _____ Reps _____ Sets _____X Day _____Hold |
|---|---|---|---|
| **13** | Notes: | **14** | Notes: |

QUAD SET –ISOMETRIC

Tighten your top thigh muscle as you attempt to press the back of your knee downward towards the table. Hold 5-10 seconds. Repeat.

Starting Position

QUAD SET WITH TOWEL UNDER HEEL - ISOMETRIC

Lying or sitting with a small towel roll under your ankle, tighten your top thigh muscle to press the back of your knee downward towards the ground. Hold 5-10 seconds. Repeat.

| | _____ Reps _____ Sets _____X Day _____Hold | | _____ Reps _____ Sets _____X Day _____Hold |
|---|---|---|---|
| **15** | Notes: | **16** | Notes: |

Starting Position

SHORT ARC QUAD (SAQ) – SELF ASSISTED

Place a rolled-up towel or other rounded object under your knee. Hook one foot under the other to assist the affected leg. Slowly straighten your knee as your raise up your foot tightening the top thigh muscle.

SHORT ARC QUAD - (SAQ) - Can add ankle weight

Place a rolled-up towel or object under your knee and slowly straighten your knee as your raise up your foot tightening the top thigh muscle. Flex your foot to increase the stretch.

# Lower Extremity Strengthening

| | _____ Reps _____ Sets _____ X Day _____ Hold | | _____ Reps _____ Sets _____ X Day _____ Hold |
|---|---|---|---|
| **17** | **Notes:** | **18** | **Notes:** |

**KNEE EXTENSION - SELF ASSISTED**

In a seated position, place the unaffected leg under the target leg. Use the unaffected leg to assist the target leg up to a straightened knee position.

**PARTIAL ARC QUAD - LOW SEAT -** Can add ankle weight

Sit with your knee in a semi bent position and your heel touching the ground and then slowly straighten your knee as you raise your foot upwards as shown. Lower your foot back down slowly controlling the muscle until your heel touches the ground and then repeat.

| | _____ Reps _____ Sets _____ X Day _____ Hold | | _____ Reps _____ Sets _____ X Day _____ Hold |
|---|---|---|---|
| **19** | **Notes:** | **20** | **Notes:** |

**LONG ARC QUAD (LAQ) – LOW SEAT (90 deg)**

Sit with your knee in a bent position and then tighten the quadricep. Slowly straighten your knee as you raise your foot upwards as shown. Lower your foot back down to original bent knee position slowly controlling the muscle and then repeat.

**LONG ARC QUAD (LAQ) – LOW SEAT - ANKLE WEIGHTS**

Attach and ankle weight. Sit with your knee in a bent position and then tighten the quadricep. Slowly straighten your knee as you raise your foot upwards as shown. Lower your foot back down to original bent knee position slowly controlling the muscle - repeat.

| | _____ Reps _____ Sets _____X Day _____Hold |
|---|---|
| **21** | **Notes:** |

LONG ARC QUAD (LAQ) - HIGH SEAT

Sit with your knee in a bent position and then tighten the quadricep. Slowly straighten your knee as you raise your foot upwards as shown. Lower your foot back down to original bent knee position slowly controlling the muscle and then repeat.

| | _____ Reps _____ Sets _____X Day _____Hold |
|---|---|
| **22** | **Notes:** |

LONG ARC QUAD (LAQ) - HIGH SEAT - ANKLE WEIGHTS

Attach and ankle weight. Sit with your knee in a bent position and then tighten the quadricep. Slowly straighten your knee as you raise your foot upwards as shown. Lower your foot back down to original bent knee position slowly controlling the muscle and then repeat.

| | _____ Reps _____ Sets _____X Day _____Hold |
|---|---|
| **23** | **Notes:** |

LONG ARC QUAD - ELASTIC BAND – HANDHELD

Attach a looped elastic band to your ankle and to the opposite foot or hold with your hand. Sit with your knee in a bent position and then tighten the quadricep. Draw your lower leg upwards to a straighten knee position while your other foot or hand secures the band. Lower your foot back down to original bent knee position slowly controlling the muscle and then repeat.

| | _____ Reps _____ Sets _____X Day _____Hold |
|---|---|
| **24** | **Notes:** |

LONG ARC QUAD - ELASTIC BAND

Attach a looped elastic band to your ankle and to a steady object behind you. Sit with your knee in a bent position and then tighten the quadricep. Draw your lower leg upwards to a straightened knee position. Lower your foot back down to original bent knee position slowly controlling the muscle and then repeat.

| | Hamstrings | | |
|---|---|---|---|

_____ Reps _____ Sets _____X Day _____Hold

**25** Notes:

_____ Reps _____ Sets _____X Day _____Hold

**26** Notes:

HAMSTRING CURLS - PRONE - ASSISTED

Lie face down and hook one foot under the other to assist the affected leg. Bend the target leg with the assistance of your unaffected leg.

HAMSTRING CURLS - PRONE

Lie face down and slowly bend your knee as you bring your foot towards your buttock.

_____ Reps _____ Sets _____X Day _____Hold

**27** Notes:

_____ Reps _____ Sets _____X Day _____Hold

**28** Notes:

HAMSTRING CURLS - - PRONE - WEIGHTS

Attach and ankle weight. Lie face down and slowly bend your knee as you bring your foot towards your buttock.

HAMSTRING CURLS – PRONE - ELASTIC BAND

Attach an elastic band around your foot and opposite ankle as shown. While lying face down, slowly bend your target knee as you bring your foot towards your buttock. Keep your other foot on the floor to fixate the band.

| | _____ Reps _____ Sets _____X Day _____Hold | | _____ Reps _____ Sets _____X Day _____Hold |
|---|---|---|---|
| **29** | **Notes:** | **30** | **Notes:** |

## HAMSTRING CURLS – ELASTIC BAND

Sit and use an elastic band secured to a steady object and the other end attached to your ankle. Bend your knee and draw back your foot.

## HAMSTRING CURLS – ELASTIC BAND - 2

Attach a looped elastic band to your ankle and to the opposite foot while one leg is propped on stool or another raised object. Draw your lower leg downwards to a bent knee position while your other ankle anchors the band on the chair.

| | _____ Reps _____ Sets _____X Day _____Hold | | _____ Reps _____ Sets _____X Day _____Hold |
|---|---|---|---|
| **31** | **Notes:** | **32** | **Notes:** **Advanced** |

## HAMSTRING CURLS ON BALL – can add ankle weight.

Lie prone on an exercise ball as shown. Slowly bend your knee as you bring your foot towards your buttock.

Starting

Position

## HAMSTRING CURLS - SINGLE LEG - EXERCISE BALL

Lie on the floor and place your heel on an exercise ball.
Lift your buttocks and then bend your knees to draw the ball towards your buttocks. Keep your buttocks elevated off the floor the entire time.

**Lower Extremity Strengthening**

## Hip Flexion

| | _____ Reps _____ Sets _____X Day _____Hold | | _____ Reps _____ Sets _____X Day _____Hold |
|---|---|---|---|
| **33** | Notes: | **34** | Notes: |

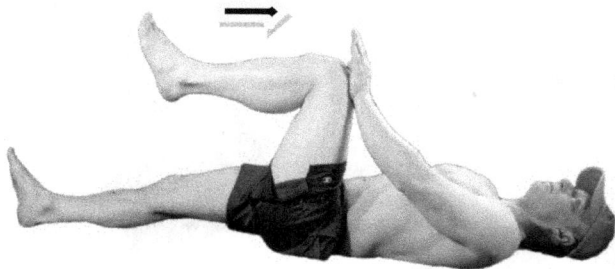

HIP FLEXION ISOMETRIC

Lie on your back, lift up your knee and press it into your hand. Hold. Return to the original position and repeat.

HIP FLEXION ISOMETRIC - ALTERNATING
Lie on your back, lift up your knee and press it into your hand. Hold. Return to the original position and repeat on the other side.

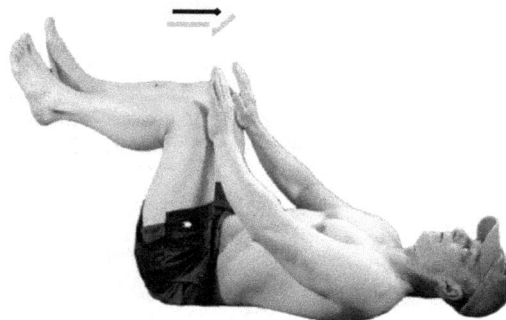

HIP FLEXION ISOMETRIC BILATERAL

Lie on your back, lift up your knees and press them into your hands. Hold. Return to the original position and repeat.

| | _____ Reps _____ Sets _____X Day _____Hold | | _____ Reps _____ Sets _____X Day _____Hold |
|---|---|---|---|
| **35** | Notes: | **36** | Notes: |

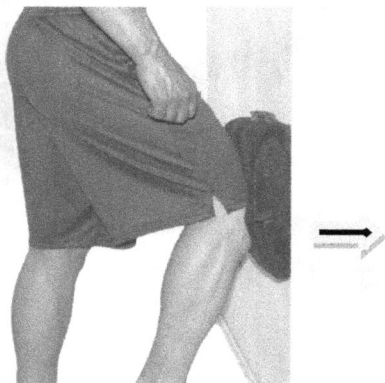

HIP FLEXION – ISOMETRIC - Can use towel roll for comfort

While standing in front of a wall, draw your knee forward and press it into the wall. Place a folded towel between your knee and the wall for comfort if needed.

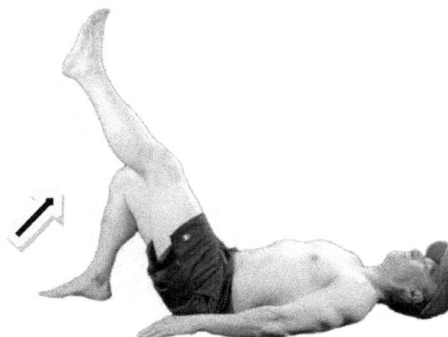

STRAIGHT LEG RAISE (SLR)

Lie on your back, tighten the quad of the target leg and lift up with a straight knee. Keep the opposite knee bent with the foot planted on the ground. (see #37 for starting position)

| | _____ Reps _____ Sets _____ X Day _____ Hold |
|---|---|
| **37** | **Notes:** |

Starting Position

STRAIGHT LEG RAISE (SLR) – ANKLE WEIGHTS

Attach ankle weights. Lie on your back and lift up your leg with a straight knee. Keep the opposite knee bent with the foot planted on the ground

| | _____ Reps _____ Sets _____ X Day _____ Hold |
|---|---|
| **38** | **Notes:** |

STRAIGHT LEG RAISE (SLR) - ELASTIC BAND

Lie on your back with an elastic band looped around your ankles, lift the target leg upwards.

| | _____ Reps _____ Sets _____ X Day _____ Hold |
|---|---|
| **39** | **Notes:** |

SEATED MARCHING - can add ankle weights for resistance

Sit in a chair and move a knee upward, set it back down and then alternate to the other side

| | _____ Reps _____ Sets _____ X Day _____ Hold |
|---|---|
| **40** | **Notes:** |

SEATED MARCHING - ELASTIC BAND

Sit in a chair with an elastic band wrapped around your thighs. Move a knee upward, set it back down and then alternate to the other side.

## Hip Extension

| | |
|---|---|
| _____ Reps _____ Sets _____X Day _____Hold | _____ Reps _____ Sets _____X Day _____Hold |
| **41**    Notes: | **42**    Notes: |

**HIP EXTENSION - PRONE**

Lie face down with your knee straight and slowly lift up leg off the ground. Maintain a straight knee the entire time.

**HIP EXTENSION – PRONE – ANKLE WEIGHTS**

Attach ankle weights. Lie face down with your knee straight and slowly lift up leg off the ground. Maintain a straight knee the entire time.

| | |
|---|---|
| _____ Reps _____ Sets _____X Day _____Hold | _____ Reps _____ Sets _____X Day _____Hold |
| **43**    Notes: | **44**    Notes: |

**HIP EXTENSION – PRONE – ELASTIC BAND**

Lie on your stomach with an elastic band looped around your ankles and lift the targeted leg upwards. Maintain a straight knee the entire time.

**HIP EXTENSION – QUADRUPED with or without ankle weights**

Start in a crawl position and then raise your leg up behind you as shown. Keep your knee bent at 90 degrees the entire time.

| **Hip Abduction (ABD)** |
|---|

_____ Reps _____ Sets _____ X Day _____ Hold

**45** Notes:

**HIP ABDUCTION - SUPINE**

Lie on your back and slowly bring your leg out to the side. Return to original position and repeat. Keep your knee straight the entire time.

_____ Reps _____ Sets _____ X Day _____ Hold

**46** Notes:

**HIP ABDUCTION - SUPINE – ANKLE WEIGHTS**

Attach and weights. Lie on your back and slowly bring your leg up slightly and then out to the side. Return to original position and repeat. Keep your knee straight the entire time.

_____ Reps _____ Sets _____ X Day _____ Hold

**47** Notes:

**HIP ABDUCTION – SUPINE - ELASTIC BAND**

Lie on your back and slowly bring your leg out to the side. Return to original position and repeat. Keep your knee straight the entire time.

_____ Reps _____ Sets _____ X Day _____ Hold

**48** Notes:

**HIP ABDUCTION / CLAMS– SUPINE - ELASTIC BAND**

Lie down on your back with your knees bent. Place an elastic band around your knees and then draw your knees apart. Return to original position and repeat.

| | _____ Reps _____ Sets _____ X Day _____ Hold |
|---|---|
| **49** | **Notes:** |

| | _____ Reps _____ Sets _____ X Day _____ Hold |
|---|---|
| **50** | **Notes:** |

MODIFIED HIP ABDUCTION – SIDELYING can add weights

Lie on your side and slowly lift up your top leg to the side. The bottom leg can be bent to stabilize your body. Keep your knee straight and maintain your toes pointed forward the entire time. Keep your leg in-line with your body. Return to original position and repeat.

HIP ABDUCTION – SIDELYING

Lie on your side and slowly lift up your top leg to the side. Keep your knee straight and maintain your toes pointed forward the entire time. Keep your leg in-line with your body. Return to original position and repeat.

| | _____ Reps _____ Sets _____ X Day _____ Hold |
|---|---|
| **51** | **Notes:** |

| | _____ Reps _____ Sets _____ X Day _____ Hold |
|---|---|
| **52** | **Notes:** |

HIP ABDUCTION – SIDELYING - WEIGHTS

Attach ankle weights. Lie on your side and slowly lift up your top leg to the side. Keep your knee straight and maintain your toes pointed forward the entire time. Keep your leg in-line with your body. Return to original position and repeat.

HIP ABDUCTION – SIDELYING - ELASTIC BAND

Lie on your side with an elastic band looped around your ankles. Lift the top leg upwards keeping your knee straight and maintaining your toes pointed forward the entire time. Keep your leg in-line with your body. Return to original position and repeat.

|  | _____ Reps _____ Sets _____ X Day _____ Hold |
|---|---|
| **53** | **Notes:** |

Starting

Position

CLAM SHELLS

Lie on your side with your knees bent, draw up the top knee while keeping contact of your feet together.
Do not let your pelvis roll back during the lifting movement.

|  | _____ Reps _____ Sets _____ X Day _____ Hold |
|---|---|
| **54** | **Notes:** |

Starting

Position

SIDELYING CLAM - ELASTIC BAND

Lie on your side with your knees bent and an elastic band wrapped around your knees, draw up the top knee while keeping contact of your feet together as shown. Do not let your pelvis roll back during the lifting movement.

|  | _____ Reps _____ Sets _____ X Day _____ Hold |
|---|---|
| **55** | **Notes:** |

Starting

Position

HIP ABDUCTION - FIRE HYDRANT - QUADRUPED

Start in a crawl position and raise your leg out to the side as shown. Maintain a straight upper and mid back.

|  | _____ Reps _____ Sets _____ X Day _____ Hold |
|---|---|
| **56** | **Notes:** |

Starting

Position

HIP ABDUCTION - FIRE HYDRANT – QUADRUPED - ELASTIC BAND

Start in a crawl position with an elastic band around your thighs. Raise your leg out to the side as shown. Maintain a straight upper and mid back.

# Lower Extremity Strengthening

| | _____ Reps _____ Sets _____X Day _____Hold |
|---|---|
| **57** | **Notes:** |

HIP ABDUCTION - SEATED - STRAIGHT LEG

Sit close to the edge of a chair with your target leg straight at the knee. Move your target leg to the side lifting slightly off the ground and then return to straight ahead.. You can slide your heel across the floor as you move and then return to straight ahead if unable to lift. Maintain your toes pointed up the entire time.

| | _____ Reps _____ Sets _____X Day _____Hold |
|---|---|
| **58** | **Notes:** |

HIP ABDUCTION - SEATED - STRAIGHT LEG – ANKLE WEIGHT

Attach an ankle weight. Sit close to the edge of a chair with your target leg straight at the knee. Move your target leg to the side lifting slightly off the ground and then return to straight ahead. Maintain your toes pointed up the entire time.

| | _____ Reps _____ Sets _____X Day _____Hold |
|---|---|
| **59** | **Notes:** |

HIP ABDUCTION - SINGLE- SEATED

Sit close to the edge of a chair with knees bent and both feet on the floor. Move your target knee out to the side as shown and then return to straight ahead. Maintain contact of your feet on the floor the entire time.

| | _____ Reps _____ Sets _____X Day _____Hold |
|---|---|
| **60** | **Notes:** |

HIP ABDUCTION - SINGLE- SEATED – ELASTIC BAND

With band tied around the thighs, sit close to the edge of a chair with knees bent and both feet on the floor. Move your target knee out to the side as shown and then return to straight ahead. Maintain contact of your feet on the floor the entire time.tact of your feet on the floor the entire time.

| _____ Reps _____ Sets _____ X Day _____ Hold |
| --- |

**61** | **Notes:**

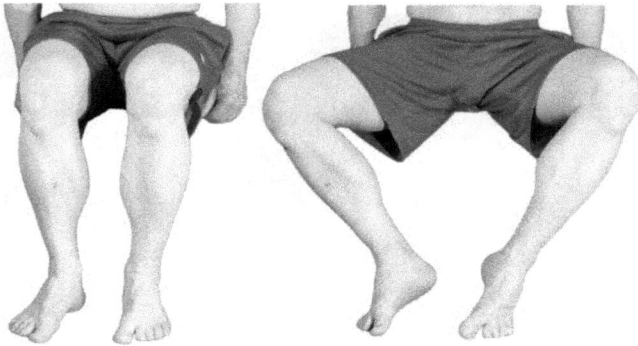

HIP ABDUCTION - BILATERAL- SEATED

Sit close to the edge of a chair with knees bent and both feet on the floor.  Move your knees out to the side as shown and then return to straight ahead. Maintain contact of your feet on the floor the entire time.

| _____ Reps _____ Sets _____ X Day _____ Hold |
| --- |

**62** | **Notes:**

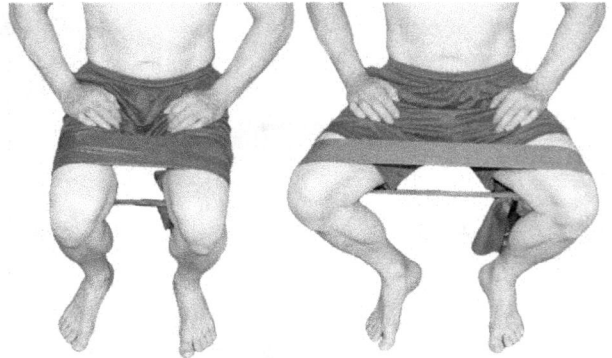

HIP ABDUCTION - BILATERAL- SEATED - ELASTIC BAND

Sit close to the edge of a chair with an elastic band wrapped around your knees.  Move both knees to the sides to separate your legs. Keep contact of your feet on the floor the entire time.

## Hip Adduction (ADD)

| _____ Reps _____ Sets _____ X Day _____ Hold |
| --- |

**63** | **Notes:**

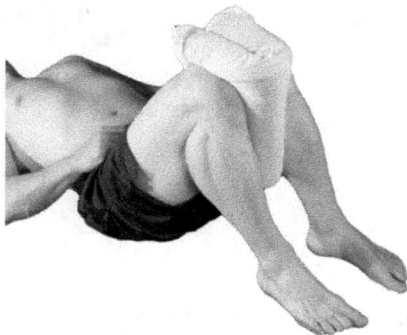

HIP ADDUCTION SQUEEZE – SUPINE – KNEES BENT

Lie on your back with legs bent and place a rolled up towel, ball or pillow between your knees. Press your knees together so that you squeeze the object firmly. Hold, release and repeat.

| _____ Reps _____ Sets _____ X Day _____ Hold |
| --- |

**64** | **Notes:**

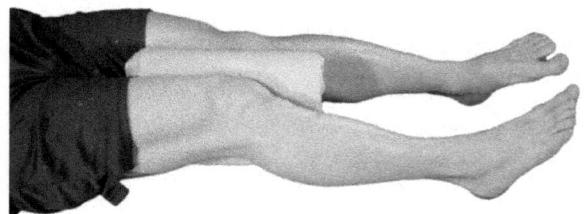

HIP ADDUCTION SQUEEZE – SUPINE – LEGS STRAIGHT

Lie on your back and place a rolled up towel, ball or pillow between your knees. Squeeze the object with your knees.  Hold, release and repeat.

| _____ Reps _____ Sets _____ X Day _____ Hold | | _____ Reps _____ Sets _____ X Day _____ Hold |
|---|---|---|
| **65** | Notes: | **66** Notes: |

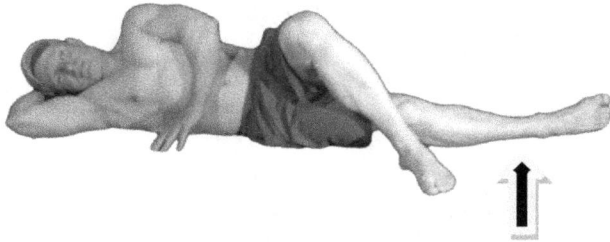

**HIP ADDUCTION - SIDELYING**

Lie on your side, slowly lift up your bottom leg towards the ceiling. Keep your knee straight the entire time. Your top leg should be bent at the knee and your foot planted on the ground supporting your body.

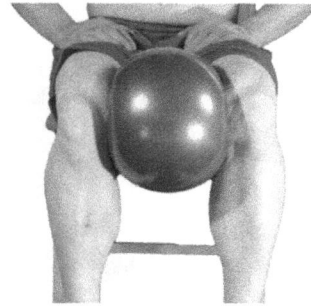

**BALL SQUEEZE - SEATED**

Sit and place a rolled-up towel, ball or pillow between your knees and squeeze the object firmly. Hold, release and repeat.

## Hip Internal Rotation (IR)

| _____ Reps _____ Sets _____ X Day _____ Hold | | _____ Reps _____ Sets _____ X Day _____ Hold |
|---|---|---|
| **67** | Notes: | **68** Notes: |

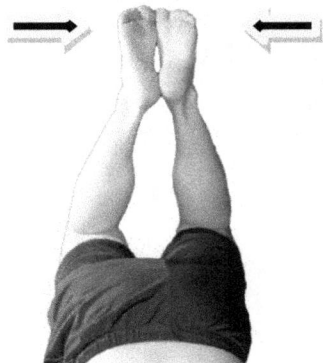

**INTERNAL ROTATION - HEEL SQUEEZE - ISOMETRIC**

Lie face down, spead your knees apart and press your heels together. Hold, release and repeat.

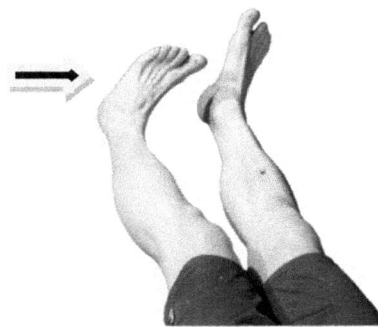

**HIP INTERNAL ROTATION - SUPINE**

Lie on your back with your knees straight, roll your hip in so that your toes point inward. Be sure that your knee cap faces inward as well.

| | _____ Reps _____ Sets _____ X Day _____ Hold |
|---|---|
| **69** | **Notes:** |

Starting
Position

REVERSE CLAMS - SIDELYING

Lie on your side with your knees bent and raise your top foot towards the ceiling while keeping contact of your knees together. Lower back down to original position. Do not let your pelvis roll forward during the lifting movement.

| | _____ Reps _____ Sets _____ X Day _____ Hold |
|---|---|
| **70** | **Notes:** |

Starting Position

REVERSE CLAMS - SIDELYING - ELASTIC BAND

Lie on your side with your knees bent and an elastic band around your ankles. Raise your top foot towards the ceiling while keeping contact of your knees together. Lower back down to original position. Do not let your pelvis roll forward during the lifting movement.

| | _____ Reps _____ Sets _____ X Day _____ Hold |
|---|---|
| **71** | **Notes:** |

HIP INTERNAL ROTATION - SEATED

Sit on a chair with your legs spread apart and feet planted on the ground. Use your hand on the inside of your knee to resist the movement inward.

| | _____ Reps _____ Sets _____ X Day _____ Hold |
|---|---|
| **72** | **Notes:** |

HIP INTERNAL ROTATION - ELASTIC BAND - High chair

Attach one end of an elastic band at your ankle and the other to a sturdy object. Pull away from your other leg while keeping your thigh from moving.

## Hip External Rotation (ER)

| | _____ Reps _____ Sets _____X Day _____Hold | | _____ Reps _____ Sets _____X Day _____Hold |
|---|---|---|---|
| **73** | **Notes:** | **74** | **Notes:** |

**HIP EXTERNAL ROTATION - SUPINE**

Lie on your back with your knees straight and roll your hip out so that your toes point outward. Be sure that your knee cap faces outward as well.

**HIP EXTERNAL ROTATION - ELASTIC BAND**

Sit and use an elastic band secured to a steady object and the other end attached to your ankle from the side.
Pull towards your other leg while keeping your thigh from moving across the table.

## Bilateral Hip Rotation

| | _____ Reps _____ Sets _____X Day _____Hold | | _____ Reps _____ Sets _____X Day _____Hold |
|---|---|---|---|
| **75** | **Notes:** | **76** | **Notes:** |

**HIP ROTATIONS – BILATERAL - SIDELYING**

Lie on your side in fetal position with knees and hips bent.
Slowly raise up both lower legs and feet as shown.
Your feet and knees should be touching the entire time.

**HIP ROTATION - SEATED - BALL and ELASTIC BAND –** High chair

Sit and place a rolled-up towel, ball or pillow between your knees and an elastic band around your ankles. Squeeze the ball, sustain and hold. Next, pull the band as you move your feet apart from each other.

## Leg Press

| | _____ Reps _____ Sets _____ X Day _____ Hold | | _____ Reps _____ Sets _____ X Day _____ Hold |
|---|---|---|---|
| **77** | Notes: | **78** | Notes: |

PRESS – BILATERAL – ELASTIC BAND

Lie on back put elastic band on bottom of both feet.  Start with knees bent and push with feet to straighten both legs.

PRESS – SINGLE LEG – ELASTIC BAND

Lie on back put elastic band on bottom of one foot.  Start with knees bent and push with foot to straighten leg.

## Hip Hikes (Gluteus Medius)

| | _____ Reps _____ Sets _____ X Day _____ Hold | | _____ Reps _____ Sets _____ X Day _____ Hold |
|---|---|---|---|
| **79** | Notes: | **80** | Notes: |

HIP HIKE -  STANDING on Step or Pad

Stand with one foot on a step or pad and the other hanging off as shown.  Raise and lower the side of your pelvis that is hanging off the edge.

HIP HIKE – KNEELING on towel or pad

Kneel on both knees with one knee on a folded towel or pad.  Raise and lower the side of your pelvis that is not on the towel/pad.

## Glutes (Glute Max)

| | \_\_\_\_\_ Reps \_\_\_\_\_ Sets \_\_\_\_\_X Day \_\_\_\_\_Hold | | \_\_\_\_\_ Reps \_\_\_\_\_ Sets \_\_\_\_\_X Day \_\_\_\_\_Hold |
|---|---|---|---|
| **81** | Notes: | **82** | Notes: |

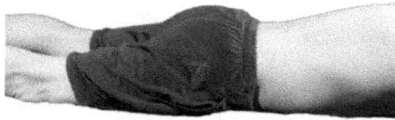

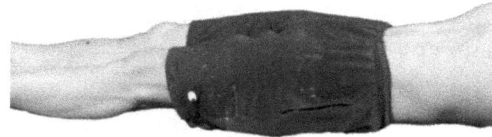

GLUTE SETS - PRONE

Lie face down, squeeze your buttocks and hold. Repeat.

GLUTE SET - SUPINE

Lie on your back, squeeze your buttocks and hold. Repeat.

| | \_\_\_\_\_ Reps \_\_\_\_\_ Sets \_\_\_\_\_X Day \_\_\_\_\_Hold | | \_\_\_\_\_ Reps \_\_\_\_\_ Sets \_\_\_\_\_X Day \_\_\_\_\_Hold |
|---|---|---|---|
| **83** | Notes: | **84** | Notes: |

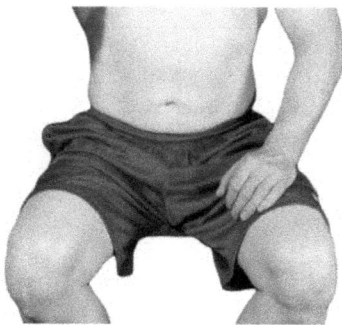

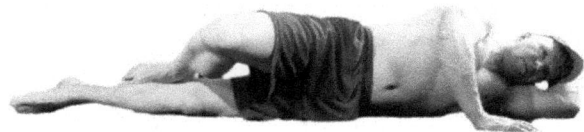

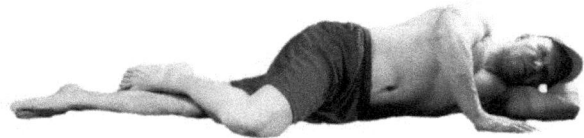

GLUTE SQUEEZE - SITTING

While sitting, squeeze your buttocks and hold. Repeat.

GLUTE SCULPT (MAX/MEDIUS)

Lie on your side leaning towards your stomach. Bend leg on target side, raise up and hold.

| EXERCISE<br><br>Upper Extremity<br>Strengthening and Range of Motion | EXERCISE<br>NUMBER | NOTES |
|---|---|---|
| ELBOW FLEXION EXTENSION - SUPINE | 1 | |
| ELBOW FLEXION / EXTENSION - GRAVITY ELIMINATED | 2 | |
| BICEPS CURLS – ALTERNATING | 3 | |
| BICEPS CURL - SELF FIXATION – ELASTIC BAND | 4 | |
| SEATED BICEPS CURLS - ALTERNATING | 5 | |
| SEATED BICEPS CURLS - BILATERAL | 6 | |
| CONCENTRATION CURLS – SITTING | 7 | |
| PREACHER CURL ON BALL | 8 | |
| BICEPS CURLS | 9 | |
| BICEPS CURLS - RADIOBRACHIALIS - HAMMER CURL | 10 | |
| BICEPS CURLS - BRACHIALIS | 11 | |
| BICEPS CURLS – ROTATE OUTWARD | 12 | |
| BICEPS CURLS – ONE ARM - ELASTIC BAND | 13 | |
| BICEPS CURLS – BILATERAL - ELASTIC BAND | 14 | |
| BICEPS CURLS - RADIOBRACHIALIS - HAMMER CURL – ONE ARM - ELASTIC BAND | 15 | |
| BICEPS CURLS - RADIOBRACHIALIS - HAMMER CURL – BILATERAL - ELASTIC BAND | 16 | |
| BICEPS CURLS – BRACHIALIS - ONE ARM - ELASTIC BAND | 17 | |
| BICEPS CURL – BRACHIALIS – BILATERAL - ELASTIC BAND | 18 | |
| TRICEPS - SELF FIXATION - ELASTIC BAND | 19 | |
| OVERHEAD TRICEPS - SELF FIXATION –SEATED OR STANDING - ELASTIC BAND | 20 | |
| TRICEP EXTENSION – SITTING OR STANDING - WEIGHT | 21 | |
| TRICEP EXTENSION – SITTING OR STANDING – BILATERAL - WEIGHT | 22 | |
| ELBOW EXTENSION - BALL | 23 | |

| EXERCISE<br><br>Upper Extremity<br>Strengthening and Range of Motion | EXERCISE<br>NUMBER | NOTES |
|---|---|---|
| ELBOW EXTENSION - SKULL CRUSHER - BALL | 24 | |
| TRICEPS - ELASTIC BAND | 25 | |
| TRICEPS - BENT OVER | 26 | |
| CHAIR DIPS / PUSH UPS | 27 | |
| DIPS OFF CHAIR | 28 | |
| PENDULUM SHOULDER FORWARD/BACK | 29 | |
| PENDULUM SHOULDER – SIDE TO SIDE | 30 | |
| PENDULUM SHOULDER CIRCLES | 31 | |
| PENDULUMS - SUPINE | 32 | |
| ISOMETRIC FLEXION | 33 | |
| SHOULDER FLEXION – SIDELYING | 34 | |
| FLEXION – SUPINE  - SINGLE OR BILATERAL | 35 | |
| FLEXION – SUPINE – SINGLE OR BILATERAL - WEIGHT | 36 | |
| FLEXION – SUPINE -  DOWEL | 37 | |
| FLEXION – SUPINE - DOWEL - Weight | 38 | |
| FLEXION - SELF FIXATION – ELASTIC BAND | 39 | |
| FLEXION – ELASTIC BAND | 40 | |
| FLEXION - STANDING - PALMS DOWN / OVERHAND DOWEL | 41 | |
| FLEXION - STANDING - PALMS UP / UNDERHAND DOWEL | 42 | |
| FLEXION – PALMS FACING INWARD | 43 | |
| FLEXION – PALMS DOWN | 44 | |
| V RAISE | 45 | |
| V RAISE – WEIGHTS | 46 | |
| MILITARY PRESS – DOWEL | 47 | |
| MILITARY PRESS - FREE WEIGHTS | 48 | |

| EXERCISE<br><br>Upper Extremity<br>Strengthening and Range of Motion | EXERCISE NUMBER | NOTES |
|---|---|---|
| ISOMETRIC EXTENSION | 49 | |
| PRONE EXTENSION - EXERCISE BALL | 50 | |
| SHOULDER EXTENSION - STANDING | 51 | |
| SHOULDER EXTENSION - STANDING - WEIGHTS | 52 | |
| EXTENSION – STANDING – DOWEL | 53 | |
| EXTENSION - SELF FIXATION - ELASTIC BAND | 54 | |
| EXTENSION - ELASTIC BAND | 55 | |
| EXTENSION - BILATERAL - ELASTIC BAND | 56 | |
| INTERNAL ROTATION – ISOMETRIC | 57 | |
| INTERNAL ROTATION - ISOMETRIC- ELEVATED | 58 | |
| INTERNAL ROTATION - SIDELYING | 59 | |
| INTERNAL ROTATION - ELASTIC BAND | 60 | |
| INTERNAL / EXTERNAL ROTATION - STANDING – DOWEL | 61 | |
| INTERNAL ROTATION – DOWEL | 62 | |
| EXTERNAL ROTATION - ISOMETRIC | 63 | |
| EXTERNAL ROTATION - ISOMETRIC – ELEVATED | 64 | |
| EXTERNAL ROTATION WITH TOWEL - SIDELYING | 65 | |
| EXTERNAL ROTATION – 90/90 - WEIGHTS | 66 | |
| EXTERNAL ROTATION - BILATERAL - ELASTIC BAND | 67 | |
| EXTERNAL ROTATION - ELASTIC BAND | 68 | |
| ADDUCTION – ISOMETRIC | 69 | |
| ADDUCTION - ELASTIC BAND | 70 | |
| ABDUCTION – ISOMETRIC | 71 | |
| HORIZONTAL ABDUCTION - DOWEL | 72 | |

| EXERCISE<br><br>Upper Extremity<br>Strengthening and Range of Motion | EXERCISE NUMBER | NOTES |
|---|---|---|
| HORIZONTAL ABDUCTION/ADDUCTTION - SUPINE | 73 | |
| HORIZONTAL ABDUCTION/ADDUCTTION - SUPINE -WEIGHT | 74 | |
| ABDUCTION - SIDELYING | 75 | |
| HORIZONTAL ABDUCTION - SIDELYING | 76 | |
| ABDUCTION – WEIGHT | 77 | |
| ABDUCTION – ELASTIC BAND | 78 | |
| HORIZONTAL ABDUCTION – BILATERAL - ELASTIC BAND | 79 | |
| 90/90 ABDUCTION - WEIGHT | 80 | |
| LATERAL RAISES | 81 | |
| LATERAL RAISES – LEAN FORWARD | 82 | |
| LATERAL RAISES – LEAN FORWARD - ARM ROTATION | 83 | |
| FRONTAL RAISE – WEIGHTS | 84 | |
| UPRIGHT ROW – WEIGHTS | 85 | |
| UPRIGHT ROW – ELASTIC BAND | 86 | |
| SHRUGS | 87 | |
| SHRUGS - WEIGHTS | 88 | |
| SHOULDER ROLLS | 89 | |
| SHOULDER ROLLS - WEIGHTS | 90 | |
| SCAPULAR RETRACTIONS - BILATERAL | 91 | |
| SCAPULAR RETRACTION – SINGLE ARM | 92 | |
| ELASTIC BAND SCAPULAR RETRACTIONS WITH MINI SHOULDER EXTENSIONS | 93 | |
| PRONE RETRACTION | 94 | |
| SCAPULAR PROTRACTION - SUPINE - BILATERAL | 95 | |
| SCAPULAR PROTRACTION - SUPINE - WEIGHT | 96 | |

| EXERCISE<br><br>Upper Extremity<br>Strengthening and Range of Motion | EXERCISE NUMBER | NOTES |
|---|---|---|
| SCAPULAR PROTRACTION - SUPINE - ELASTIC BAND | 97 | |
| SCAPULAR PROTRACTION / TABLE PLANK | 98 | |
| CHEST PRESS – SEATED or STANDING - ELASTIC BAND | 99 | |
| CHEST PRESS – BALL, FLOOR or BENCH- WEIGHTS | 100 | |
| DOWEL PRESS – STANDING | 101 | |
| CHEST PRESS – STANDING or SEATED | 102 | |
| BENT OVER ROWS | 103 | |
| ROWS – PRONE | 104 | |
| ROWS - ELASTIC BAND | 105 | |
| WIDE ROWS - ELASTIC BAND | 106 | |
| LOW ROW – ELASTIC BAND | 107 | |
| HIGH ROW – ELASTIC BAND | 108 | |
| FLY'S – FLOOR - WEIGHT | 109 | |
| FLY'S – BALL or BENCH – WEIGHT | 110 | |
| WALL PUSH UPS | 111 | |
| WALL PUSH UP - BALL | 112 | |
| WALL PUSH UP - Triceps uneven | 113 | |
| WALL PUSH UP - Hands inverted | 114 | |
| WALL PUSH UP - Narrow | 115 | |
| WALL PUSH UP – Wide | 116 | |
| PUSH UPS - BALL | 117 | |
| PUSH UP - MODIFIED | 118 | |
| PUSH UP | 119 | |
| PUSH UP -DIAMOND | 120 | |
| PUSH UP – MODIFIED - BOSU - UNSTABLE | 121 | |

| EXERCISE<br><br>Upper Extremity<br>Strengthening and Range of Motion | EXERCISE<br>NUMBER | NOTES |
|---|---|---|
| PUSH UP – BOSU - UNSTABLE | 122 | |
| PUSH UP – MODIFIED – INVERTED BOSU - UNSTABLE | 123 | |
| PUSH UP – INVERTED BOSU - UNSTABLE | 124 | |

# UPPER EXTREMITY - Range Of Motion > Isometric > Strength

## Elbow Flexion/Extension

| | | | |
|---|---|---|---|
| | _____ Reps _____ Sets _____ X Day _____ Hold | | _____ Reps _____ Sets _____ X Day _____ Hold |
| **1** | Notes: | **2** | Notes: |

ELBOW FLEXION EXTENSION - SUPINE

Lie on your back and rest your elbow on a small rolled up towel. Bend at your elbow and then lower back down.

ELBOW FLEXION / EXTENSION - GRAVITY ELIMINATED

Sit and hold your arm up with the help of your other arm. Bend and straighten your elbow.

## Elbow Flexion (Biceps)

| | | | |
|---|---|---|---|
| | _____ Reps _____ Sets _____ X Day _____ Hold | | _____ Reps _____ Sets _____ X Day _____ Hold |
| **3** | Notes: | **4** | Notes: |

BICEPS CURLS – ALTERNATING

Bend your elbow and move your forearm upwards. As you lower back down, begin bending the opposite elbow upwards.

BICEPS CURL - SELF FIXATION – ELASTIC BAND

Sit and hold an elastic band with one hand. Hold the other end of elastic band with the opposite hand and fixate hand on your knee. Slowly draw up your hand by bending at the elbow. Return to starting position and repeat.

*Can increase resistance by doubling band as shown.

| | _____ Reps _____ Sets _____X Day _____Hold | | _____ Reps _____ Sets _____X Day _____Hold |
|---|---|---|---|
| **5** | **Notes:** | **6** | **Notes:** |

SEATED BICEPS CURLS - ALTERNATING

Sit in a chair and hold free weights on each thigh. Lift one side while bending at the elbow and squeezing bicep muscle. Perform on one side and then alternate to the other side.

SEATED BICEPS CURLS - BILATERAL

Sit in a chair and hold free weights on each thigh. Lift both sides while bending at the elbows and squeezing bicep muscles. Lower back down and repeat.

| | _____ Reps _____ Sets _____X Day _____Hold | | _____ Reps _____ Sets _____X Day _____Hold |
|---|---|---|---|
| **7** | **Notes:** | **8** | **Notes:** |

Starting Position

CONCENTRATION CURLS – SITTING

Sit in a chair, lean slightly forward and hold a free weight with arm straight with elbow on inside of thigh. Bend elbow squeezing bicep muscle. Lower back down - repeat.

PREACHER CURL ON BALL

Lie on stomach over ball in crawling position. Hold weights in both hands with back of arms against ball. Lift both sides while bending at the elbows and squeezing bicep muscles. Lower back down - repeat.

| 9 | _____ Reps _____ Sets _____ X Day _____ Hold <br><br> Notes: | 10 | _____ Reps _____ Sets _____ X Day _____ Hold <br><br> Notes: |
|---|---|---|---|

BICEPS CURLS

Holding weights and keeping your arm at your side, draw up your hand by bending at the elbow squeezing bicep muscle.  Keep your palm face up the entire time.  Can perform set on one side and then other or alternate arms.

BICEPS CURLS - RADIOBRACHIALIS - HAMMER CURL

Holding weights and keeping your arm at your side, draw up your hand by bending at the elbow squeezing bicep muscle.  Keep your wrist in a neutral position as shown above the entire time.  Can perform set on one side and then other or alternate arms.

| 11 | _____ Reps _____ Sets _____ X Day _____ Hold <br><br> Notes: | 12 | _____ Reps _____ Sets _____ X Day _____ Hold <br><br> Notes: |
|---|---|---|---|

BICEPS CURLS - BRACHIALIS

Holding weights and keeping your arm at your side, draw up your hand by bending at the elbow squeezing bicep muscle. Keep your palm face down the entire time.  Can perform set on one side and then other or alternate arms.

BICEPS CURLS – ROTATE OUTWARD

Holding weights and keeping your arm at your side, draw up your hand by bending at the elbow squeezing bicep muscle. Keep your palm face up the entire time.  You can do this one arm at a time or bilateral.

| | _____ Reps _____ Sets _____X Day _____Hold | | _____ Reps _____ Sets _____X Day _____Hold |
|---|---|---|---|
| **13** | **Notes:** | **14** | **Notes:** |

**BICEPS CURLS – ONE ARM - ELASTIC BAND**

In a standing position, step on the band with one leg. Keep your arm at your side holding an elastic band and draw up your hand by bending at the elbow squeezing bicep muscle. Keep your palm face up the entire time.

**BICEPS CURLS – BILATERAL - ELASTIC BAND**

In a standing position, step on the band with both feet, shoulder width apart. Keep your arms at your side holding an elastic band and draw up your hands by bending at the elbows squeezing bicep muscles. Keep your palms facing upward the entire time.

| | _____ Reps _____ Sets _____X Day _____Hold | | _____ Reps _____ Sets _____X Day _____Hold |
|---|---|---|---|
| **15** | **Notes:** | **16** | **Notes:** |

**BICEPS CURLS - RADIOBRACHIALIS - HAMMER CURL – ONE ARM - ELASTIC BAND**

In a standing position, step on the band with one leg. Keep your arm at your side holding an elastic band and draw up your hand by bending at the elbow squeezing bicep muscle. Keep your palm facing inward the entire time.

**BICEPS CURLS - RADIOBRACHIALIS - HAMMER CURL – BILATERAL - ELASTIC BAND**

In a standing position, step on the band with both feet, shoulder width apart. Keep your arms at your side holding an elastic band and draw up your hands by bending at the elbows squeezing bicep muscles. Keep your palms facing inward the entire time.

| | _____ Reps _____ Sets _____ X Day _____ Hold |
|---|---|
| **17** | **Notes:** |

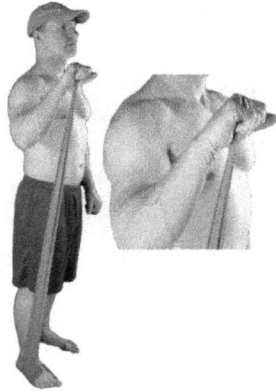

BICEPS CURLS – BRACHIALIS - ONE ARM - ELASTIC BAND

In a standing position, step on the band with one leg. Keep your arm at your side holding an elastic band and draw up your hand by bending at the elbow squeezing bicep muscle. Keep your palm face down the entire time.

| | _____ Reps _____ Sets _____ X Day _____ Hold |
|---|---|
| **18** | **Notes:** |

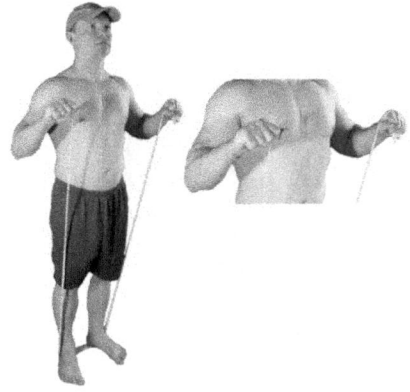

BICEPS CURL – BRACHIALIS – BILATERAL - ELASTIC BAND

In a standing position, step on the band with both feet, shoulder width apart. Keep your arms at your side holding an elastic band and draw up your hands by bending at the elbows squeezing bicep muscles. Keep your palms facing downward the entire time.

## Elbow Extension (Triceps)

| | _____ Reps _____ Sets _____ X Day _____ Hold |
|---|---|
| **19** | **Notes:** |

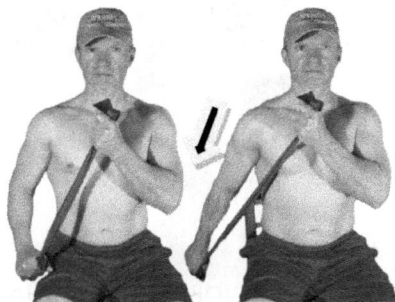

TRICEPS - SELF FIXATION - ELASTIC BAND

Hold an elastic band across your chest with the unaffected arm. Pull the band downward with the other arm so that the elbow goes from a bent position to a straightened position as shown.

| | _____ Reps _____ Sets _____ X Day _____ Hold |
|---|---|
| **20** | **Notes:** |

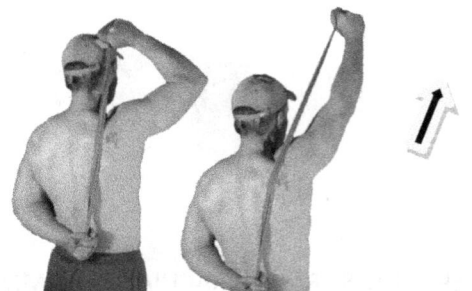

OVERHEAD TRICEPS - SELF FIXATION –SEATED OR STANDING - ELASTIC BAND

Hold an elastic band with one arm fixated behind back as shown and other hand behind head. Extend elbow with arm overhead and return to starting position.

| | _____ Reps _____ Sets _____ X Day _____ Hold | | | _____ Reps _____ Sets _____ X Day _____ Hold |
|---|---|---|---|---|
| **21** | **Notes:** | | **22** | **Notes:** |

TRICEP EXTENSION – SITTING OR STANDING - WEIGHT

Start with hand behind head holding free weight. Extend your elbow as shown. Maintain your upper arm in an upward direction and only bend and straighten at your elbow.
*Can hold the triceps area with opposite arm to stabilize.

TRICEP EXTENSION – SITTING OR STANDING – BILATERAL - WEIGHT

Start with hands behind head holding free weight Extend your elbows while holding a free weight in both hands. Maintain your upper arms in an upward direction and only bend and straighten at your elbows.

| | _____ Reps _____ Sets _____ X Day _____ Hold | | | _____ Reps _____ Sets _____ X Day _____ Hold |
|---|---|---|---|---|
| **23** | **Notes:** | | **24** | **Notes:** |

ELBOW EXTENSION - BALL

Lie on your back on ball. Extend your elbow as shown while holding a free weight in each hand. Maintain your upper arms in an upward direction and only bend and straighten at your elbows.

ELBOW EXTENSION - SKULL CRUSHER - BALL

Lie on your back on ball with a free weight in each hand. Bend your elbows to lower the weight towards the side of your head and then extend arms straight up towards the ceiling.

| | | | |
|---|---|---|---|
| | _____ Reps _____ Sets _____X Day _____Hold | | _____ Reps _____ Sets _____X Day _____Hold |
| **25** | Notes: | **26** | Notes: |

**TRICEPS - ELASTIC BAND**

Fixate the band at top of door. Start with your elbow bent and holding an elastic band as shown. Pull the elastic band downward as you extend your elbow. Keep your elbow by your side the entire time.

**TRICEPS - BENT OVER**

Stand and bend over with either support or placing your unaffected arm on thigh for support. With your targeted arm and elbow at your side, extend your elbow as you straighten your arm as shown. Keep your elbow at your side and back flat the entire time.

| | | | |
|---|---|---|---|
| | _____ Reps _____ Sets _____X Day _____Hold | | _____ Reps _____ Sets _____X Day _____Hold |
| **27** | Notes: | **28** | Notes: |

**CHAIR DIPS / PUSH UPS**

While sitting in a chair with arm rests, push yourself upawards so that you lift your buttocks of the chair and then lower down controlled back to normal seated position. *If you are unable to lift yourself up, you can perform "pressure releases" so that you simply push to take some weight off your buttocks.

**DIPS OFF CHAIR**

Push yourself up to a straight elbow position as shown. Then lower your buttocks down towards the floor by bending your elbows.

## Shoulder PENDULUMS

| | _____ Reps _____ Sets _____ X Day _____ Hold | | _____ Reps _____ Sets _____ X Day _____ Hold |
|---|---|---|---|
| **29** | Notes: | **30** | Notes: |

**PENDULUM SHOULDER FORWARD/BACK**

Shift your body weight forward then back to allow your injured arm to swing forward and back freely. Your affected arm should be fully relaxed.

**PENDULUM SHOULDER – SIDE TO SIDE**

Shift your body weight side to side to allow your injured arm to swing side to side freely. Your affected arm should be fully relaxed.

| | _____ Reps _____ Sets _____ X Day _____ Hold | | _____ Reps _____ Sets _____ X Day _____ Hold |
|---|---|---|---|
| **31** | Notes: | **32** | Notes: |

**PENDULUM SHOULDER CIRCLES**
Shift your body weight in circles to allow your injured arm to swing in circles freely. Your injured arm should be fully relaxed.
**REVERSE PENDULUM SHOULDER CIRCLES**
Shift your body weight into reverse circles to allow your injured arm to swing in circles freely. Your injured arm should be fully relaxed.

**PENDULUMS - SUPINE**

Lie on your back and straighten your arm towards the ceiling. Move your arm in small circles in a clockwise motion. After a few seconds, reverse the direction to a counterclockwise motion. Change directions every few seconds.

## Shoulder Flexion

| | _____ Reps _____ Sets _____X Day _____Hold | | _____ Reps _____ Sets _____X Day _____Hold |
|---|---|---|---|
| **33** | Notes: | **34** | Notes: |

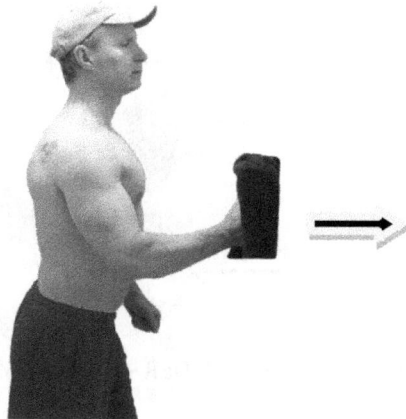

ISOMETRIC FLEXION - Can use towel roll for comfort

Gently push your fist forward into a wall with your elbow bent. Hold for 5-10 seconds. Repeat.

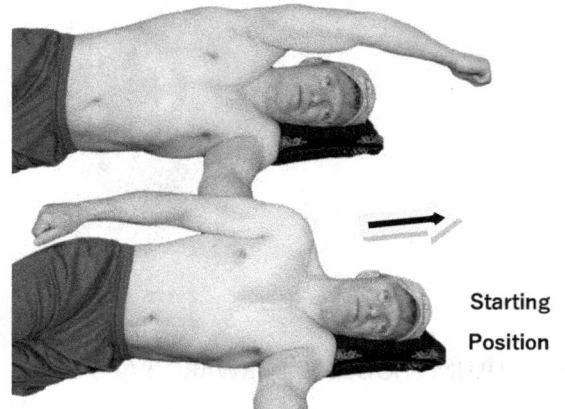

SHOULDER FLEXION – SIDELYING - Can add weight

Lie on your side with arm at your side. Slowly raise the arm forward towards overhead and in front of your body.

| | _____ Reps _____ Sets _____X Day _____Hold | | _____ Reps _____ Sets _____X Day _____Hold |
|---|---|---|---|
| **35** | Notes: | **36** | Notes: |

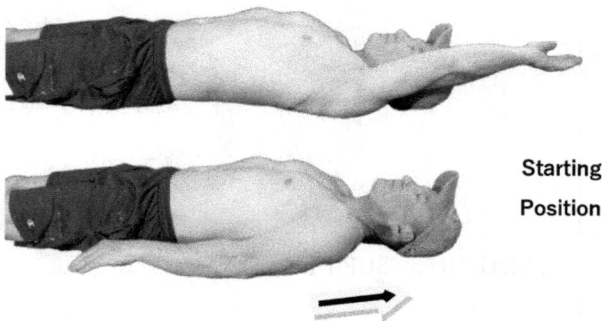

FLEXION – SUPINE - SINGLE OR BILATERAL

Lie on your back with your arm at your side. Slowly raise arm up and forward towards overhead.

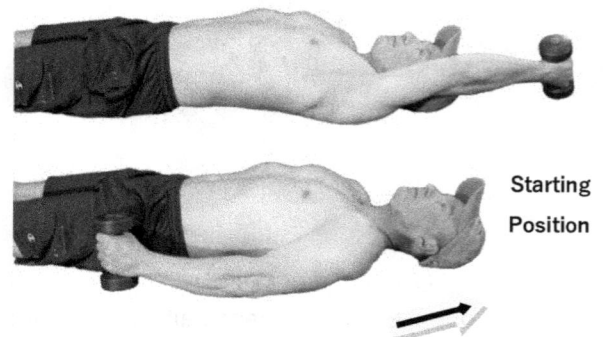

FLEXION – SUPINE – SINGLE OR BILATERAL - WEIGHT

Lie on your back with your arm at your side. Holding a weight, slowly raise arm up and forward towards overhead.

| _____ Reps _____ Sets _____X Day _____Hold | | _____ Reps _____ Sets _____X Day _____Hold | |
|---|---|---|---|
| **37** | **Notes:** | **38** | **Notes:** |

Starting Position

Starting Position

FLEXION – SUPINE - DOWEL

Lie on your back holding dowel with both hands. Slowly raise up and forward towards overhead. Return to starting position. Repeat.
*If you have an injury/weakness, allow your unaffected arm to perform most of the effort. Your affected arm should be partially relaxed.

FLEXION – SUPINE - DOWEL – Add weight only if equal strength

Attach ankle weight to dowel. Lie on your back holding dowel with both hands. Slowly raise up and forward towards overhead. Return to starting position. Repeat.

| _____ Reps _____ Sets _____X Day _____Hold | | _____ Reps _____ Sets _____X Day _____Hold | |
|---|---|---|---|
| **39** | **Notes:** | **40** | **Notes:** |

Starting Position

FLEXION - SELF FIXATION – ELASTIC BAND

Hold an elastic band in front and fixate unaffected arm straight by your side or on your leg. Pull the band upward towards the ceiling with your target arm.

FLEXION – ELASTIC BAND

In a standing position, step on the band with one leg. Keep your arm at your side holding an elastic band and draw up your arm up in front of you keeping your elbow straight.

| _____ Reps _____ Sets _____X Day _____Hold | | _____ Reps _____ Sets _____X Day _____Hold |
|---|---|---|

**41** Notes:

**42** Notes:

FLEXION - STANDING - PALMS DOWN / OVERHAND DOWEL - Add weight only if equal strength

Hold a dowel/cane with both arms, palm down on both sides. Raise the dowel forward and up. (see #39/40) *Do not use weight if you have an injury/weakness. Allow your unaffected arm to perform most of the work. Your affected arm should be partially relaxed.

FLEXION - STANDING - PALMS UP /UNDERHAND DOWEL - Add weight only if equal strength

Hold a dowel/cane with both arms and palms up on both sides. Raise the dowel forward and up. *Do not use weight if you have an injury/weakness. Allow your unaffected arm to perform most of the work. Your affected arm should be partially relaxed.

| _____ Reps _____ Sets _____X Day _____Hold | | _____ Reps _____ Sets _____X Day _____Hold |
|---|---|---|

**43** Notes:

**44** Notes:

FLEXION – PALMS FACING INWARD - Can remove weight BILATERAL or ALTERNATE ARMS.

Sit or stand with your arm at your side. Hold a free weight with your palm facing your side and your elbows straight. Raise up your arm forward as shown then return to starting position. Do not let your shoulder shrug upwards unless instructed to go over shoulder level height.

FLEXION – PALMS DOWN - Can remove weight BILATERAL or ALTERNATE ARMS.

Sit or stand with your arm at your side. Hold a weight with your palm facing down and your elbows straight. Raise up your arm forward as shown then return to starting position. Do not let your shoulder shrug upwards unless instructed to go over shoulder height.

## V Raises

| 45 | _____ Reps _____ Sets _____ X Day _____ Hold |  | 46 | _____ Reps _____ Sets _____ X Day _____ Hold |
|---|---|---|---|---|
| | Notes: | | | Notes: |

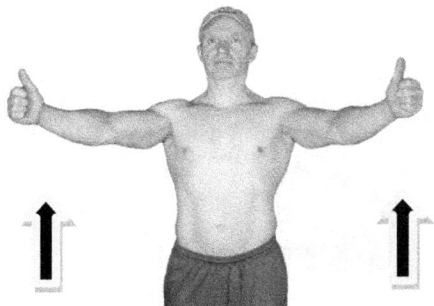

V RAISE

Start with your arms down by your side, palms facing inward, thumbs up and your elbows straight. Raise up your arms in the form of a V to shoulder height as shown keeping elbows straight then return to starting position.

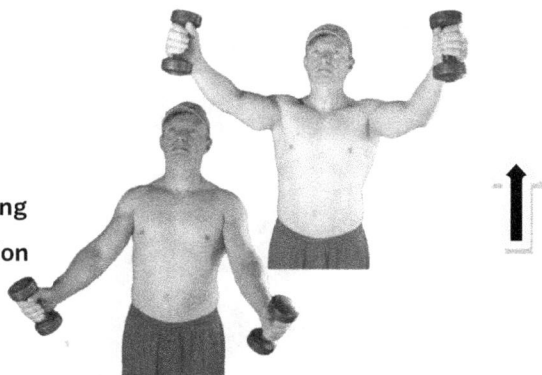

Starting Position

V RAISE – WEIGHTS

Holding free weights, start with your arms down by your side, palms facing inward and your elbows straight. Raise up your arms in the form of a V to shoulder height keeping elbows straight – return.

## Shoulder Press

| 47 | _____ Reps _____ Sets _____ X Day _____ Hold |  | 48 | _____ Reps _____ Sets _____ X Day _____ Hold |
|---|---|---|---|---|
| | Notes: | | | Notes: |

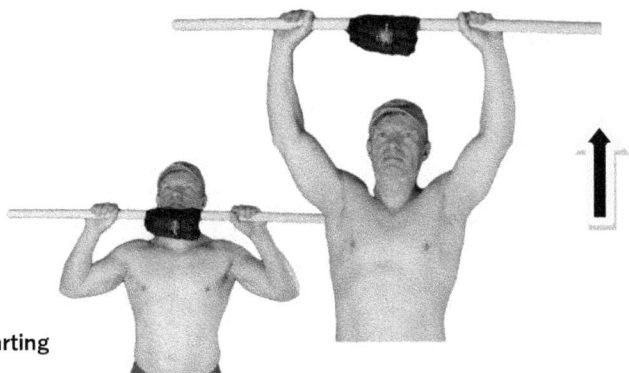

Starting Position

MILITARY PRESS – DOWEL- Add weight only if equal strength

Hold a dowel or cane at chest height. Slowly push the wand upwards towards the ceiling until your elbows become fully straightened. Return to the original position.

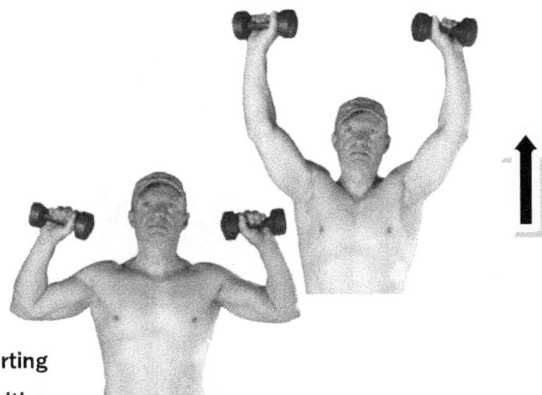

Starting Position

MILITARY PRESS - FREE WEIGHTS

Hold free weights at 90-degree angle as shown above.
Slowly push your arms upwards towards the ceiling until your elbows become fully straightened. Return to the original position.

## Shoulder Extension

| | |
|---|---|
| _____ Reps _____ Sets _____ X Day _____ Hold | _____ Reps _____ Sets _____ X Day _____ Hold |
| **49**   Notes: | **50**   Notes: |

ISOMETRIC EXTENSION - Can use towel roll for comfort

Gently push your bent elbow back into a wall. Hold for 5-10 seconds. Relax and repeat.

PRONE EXTENSION - EXERCISE BALL – Can add weights.

Lie face down over an exercise ball with your elbows straight and along the side of your body. Slowly raise your arms upward along your side and then return to original position.

| | |
|---|---|
| _____ Reps _____ Sets _____ X Day _____ Hold | _____ Reps _____ Sets _____ X Day _____ Hold |
| **51**   Notes: | **52**   Notes: |

SHOULDER EXTENSION - STANDING

Start with arms by your side. Draw your arm back behind your waist. Keep your elbows straight.

SHOULDER EXTENSION - STANDING - WEIGHTS

Hold a weight by your side and draw your arm back. Keep your elbows straight.

| | _____ Reps _____ Sets _____X Day _____Hold |
|---|---|
| **53** | **Notes:** |

Starting

Position

EXTENSION – STANDING – DOWEL - Add weight only if equal strength

Hold a dowel or cane behind your back with both arms. Draw your arms back.

| | _____ Reps _____ Sets _____X Day _____Hold |
|---|---|
| **54** | **Notes:** |

EXTENSION - SELF FIXATION - ELASTIC BAND

Hold an elastic band out in front of you with your fixated arm. Pull the band downward towards the ground and backwards with your target arm.

| | _____ Reps _____ Sets _____X Day _____Hold |
|---|---|
| **55** | **Notes:** |

EXTENSION - ELASTIC BAND

Fixate the end of an elastic band at top of door. Hold the elastic band in front of you with your elbows straight. Slowly pull the band down and back towards your side.

| | _____ Reps _____ Sets _____X Day _____Hold |
|---|---|
| **56** | **Notes:** |

EXTENSION - BILATERAL - ELASTIC BAND

Fixate the middle of an elastic band at top of door. Hold the elastic band with both arms in front of you with your elbows straight. Slowly pull the band downwards and back towards your side.

# Shoulder Internal Rotation (IR)

| | _____ Reps _____ Sets _____ X Day _____ Hold | | _____ Reps _____ Sets _____ X Day _____ Hold |
|---|---|---|---|
| **57** | **Notes:** | **58** | **Notes:** |

INTERNAL ROTATION – ISOMETRIC - Can use towel roll for comfort

Press your hand into a wall using the palm side of your hand and hold.  Maintain a bent elbow the entire time.

INTERNAL ROTATION - ISOMETRIC- ELEVATED - Can use towel roll for comfort

Push the front of your hand into a wall with your elbow bent and arm elevated and hold.

| | _____ Reps _____ Sets _____ X Day _____ Hold | | _____ Reps _____ Sets _____ X Day _____ Hold |
|---|---|---|---|
| **59** | **Notes:** | **60** | **Notes:** |

INTERNAL ROTATION - SIDELYING

Lie on your side with your shoulder flexed to 90 degrees and elbow bent and rested on the table/bed/matt. Your forearm should be pointing up towards the ceiling. Allow your forearm to lower toward the table as shown. Place a rolled-up towel under your elbow if needed.

INTERNAL ROTATION - ELASTIC BAND

Hold an elastic band at your side with your elbow bent. Start with your hand away from your stomach and then pull the band towards your stomach. Keep your elbow near your side the entire time.

| | _____ Reps _____ Sets _____ X Day _____ Hold |
|---|---|
| **61** | **Notes:** |

INTERNAL / EXTERNAL ROTATION - STANDING – DOWEL
Add weight only if equal strength

Stand and hold a dowel/cane with both hands keeping your elbows bent. Move your arms and dowel/cane side-to-side. _If you have an injury/weakness, the affected arm should be partially relaxed while your unaffected arm performs most of the effort._

| | _____ Reps _____ Sets _____ X Day _____ Hold |
|---|---|
| **62** | **Notes:** |

Starting Position

INTERNAL ROTATION – DOWEL - Add weight only if equal strength

While holding a dowel/cane behind your back, slowly pull the wand up.

## Shoulder External Rotation (ER)

| | _____ Reps _____ Sets _____ X Day _____ Hold |
|---|---|
| **63** | **Notes:** |

EXTERNAL ROTATION - ISOMETRIC – Can use towel roll for comfort

Gently press your hand into a wall using the back side of your hand. Maintain a bent elbow the entire time.

| | _____ Reps _____ Sets _____ X Day _____ Hold |
|---|---|
| **64** | **Notes:** |

EXTERNAL ROTATION - ISOMETRIC – ELEVATED - Can use towel roll for comfort

Gently push the back of your hand/arm into a wall with your arm elevated.

| _____ Reps _____ Sets _____ X Day _____ Hold |
| --- |

| 65 | Notes: |
| --- | --- |

EXTERNAL ROTATION WITH TOWEL - SIDELYING

Lie on your side with your elbow bent to 90 degrees. Place a rolled-up towel between your arm and the side your body as shown. Squeeze your shoulder blade back and rotate arm up and hold this position. Slowly rotate back to original position and repeat.

| _____ Reps _____ Sets _____ X Day _____ Hold |
| --- |

| 66 | Notes: |
| --- | --- |

EXTERNAL ROTATION – 90/90 - WEIGHTS

Hold weights with elbows bent to 90 degrees and away from your side. Rotate your shoulders back so that the palms of your hands face forward and then return as shown.

| _____ Reps _____ Sets _____ X Day _____ Hold |
| --- |

| 67 | Notes: |
| --- | --- |

EXTERNAL ROTATION - BILATERAL - ELASTIC BAND
Can put a towel between side and elbow (see #68)

Hold an elastic band with your elbows bent, pull your hands away from your stomach area. Keep your elbows near the side of your body.

| _____ Reps _____ Sets _____ X Day _____ Hold |
| --- |

| 68 | Notes: |
| --- | --- |

EXTERNAL ROTATION - ELASTIC BAND – Can add roll between side and arm

Fixate an elastic band to the door at elbow height. Hold the other end of the band at your side with your elbow bent. Start with your hand near your stomach and then pull the band away. Keep your elbow at your side the entire time.

## Shoulder Adduction (ADD)

| | |
|---|---|
| _____ Reps _____ Sets _____X Day _____Hold | _____ Reps _____ Sets _____X Day _____Hold |
| **69** Notes: | **70** Notes: |

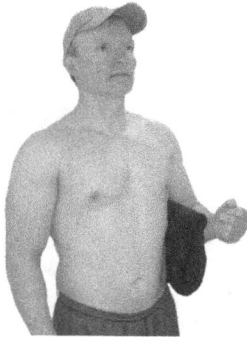

ADDUCTION – ISOMETRIC - Can use towel roll for comfort

Place a towel roll between your bent elbow and body. Gently push your elbow into the side of your body.

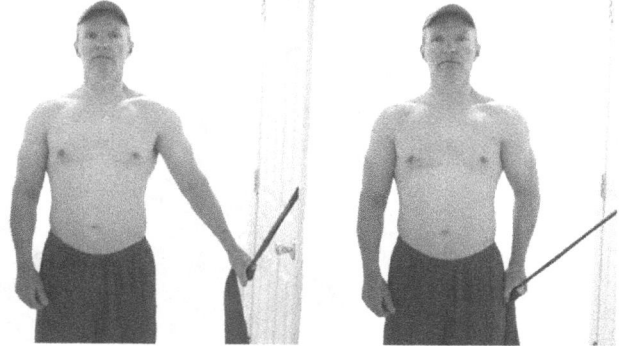

ADDUCTION - ELASTIC BAND

Fixate an elastic band to the door and hold the other end of the band away from your side. Pull the band towards your side keeping your elbow straight.

## Shoulder Abduction (ABD)

| | |
|---|---|
| _____ Reps _____ Sets _____X Day _____Hold | _____ Reps _____ Sets _____X Day _____Hold |
| **71** Notes: | **72** Notes: |

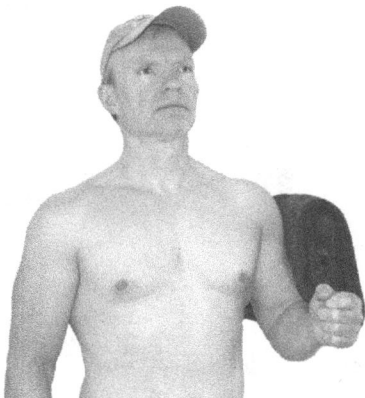

ABDUCTION – ISOMETRIC - Can use towel roll for comfort

Gently push your elbow out to the side into a wall with your elbow bent.

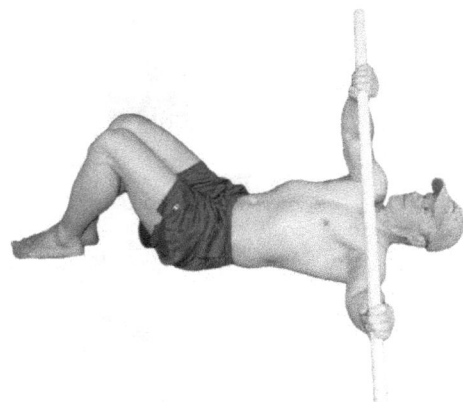

HORIZONTAL ABDUCTION - DOWEL

Lie on your back holding a dowel/cane straight up towards the ceiling with your elbows straight. Bring your arms and wand to the side and then towards the other.

| | | |
|---|---|---|
| | _____ Reps _____ Sets _____X Day _____Hold | _____ Reps _____ Sets _____X Day _____Hold |
| **73** | Notes: | |
| **74** | Notes: | |

**HORIZONTAL ABDUCTION/ADDUCTTION - SUPINE**
Lie on your back with arm straight up in front of your body. Slowly lower your arm out towards the side. Return to original position.

**HORIZONTAL ABDUCTION/ADDUCTTION - SUPINE - WEIGHT**

Hold a weight. Lie on your back with arm straight up in front of your body. Slowly lower your arm out towards the side. Return to original position

| | | |
|---|---|---|
| | _____ Reps _____ Sets _____X Day _____Hold | _____ Reps _____ Sets _____X Day _____Hold |
| **75** | Notes: | |
| **76** | Notes: | |

**ABDUCTION - SIDELYING - Can add weight**

Lie on your side with arm at your side. Slowly raise the target arm up towards head and away from your side.

**HORIZONTAL ABDUCTION - SIDELYING - Can add weight**

Lie on your side with arm out in front of your body. Slowly raise up the arm overhead towards the ceiling.

| | _____ Reps _____ Sets _____X Day _____Hold | | _____ Reps _____ Sets _____X Day _____Hold |
|---|---|---|---|
| **77** | **Notes:** | **78** | **Notes:** |

**ABDUCTION – WEIGHT – Can do without a weight**

Hold a weight with your affected arm at your side. Keeping your elbow straight, raise up your arm to the side.

**ABDUCTION – ELASTIC BAND**

Fixate an elastic band under a door and hold band with hand farthest away from door at your side. Keeping your elbow straight, raise up your arm to the side.

| | _____ Reps _____ Sets _____X Day _____Hold | | _____ Reps _____ Sets _____X Day _____Hold |
|---|---|---|---|
| **79** | **Notes:** | **80** | **Notes:** |

**HORIZONTAL ABDUCTION – BILATERAL - ELASTIC BAND**

Hold an elastic band in both hands with your elbows straight in front of your body. Slowly pull your arms apart towards the sides.

**90/90 ABDUCTION - WEIGHT**

Hold weights at your side with elbows bent to 90 degrees. Raise up your elbows away from your side while maintaining your elbows bent at 90 degrees.

# Lateral/Frontal Raise

| | _____ Reps _____ Sets _____X Day _____Hold |
|---|---|
| **81** | **Notes:** |

Starting Position

LATERAL RAISES

Hold weights at your side with arms straight. Raise up your elbows away from your side while keeping your elbow straight the entire time.

| | _____ Reps _____ Sets _____X Day _____Hold |
|---|---|
| **82** | **Notes:** |

Starting Position

LATERAL RAISES – LEAN FORWARD

Bend slightly at the waist holding weights slightly in front. Raise up your elbows away from your side squeezing shoulder blades together.

| | _____ Reps _____ Sets _____X Day _____Hold |
|---|---|
| **83** | **Notes:** |

Starting Position

LATERAL RAISES – LEAN FORWARD - ARM ROTATION

Bend slightly at the waist holding weights slightly in front as shown palms facing your body.  Raise up your elbows away from your side squeezing shoulder blades together.

| | _____ Reps _____ Sets _____X Day _____Hold |
|---|---|
| **84** | **Notes:** |

FRONTAL RAISE – WEIGHTS – Can do without weights

Hold weights at your side with arms straight. Slowly raise your arms in front of of your body.

## Upright Rows

| _____ Reps _____ Sets _____ X Day _____ Hold | | _____ Reps _____ Sets _____ X Day _____ Hold |
|---|---|---|

**85** Notes:

**86** Notes:

UPRIGHT ROW – WEIGHTS - Can use kettle bell

Hold weights or kettlebell with both hands at waist height. Lift the weights to chest height as you bend at your elbows.

UPRIGHT ROW – ELASTIC BAND

Stand on an elastic band with either one or both feet. Hold band at waist height and raise it up to chest height as you bend at your elbows.

## Shoulder Shrugs & Rolls

**87** Notes:

**88** Notes:

_____ Reps _____ Sets _____ X Day _____ Hold

SHRUGS

Raise your shoulders upward towards your ears as shown. Shrug both shoulders at the same time.

SHRUGS - WEIGHTS

Hold weights in both hands with arms straight. Raise your shoulders upward towards your ears. Shrug both shoulders at the same time.

| | _____ Reps _____ Sets _____X Day _____Hold |
|---|---|
| **89** | **Notes:** |

SHOULDER ROLLS

Move your shoulders in a circular pattern so that your are moving in an up, back and down direction. Perform small circles if needed for comfort.
Complete one set and then reverse direction

| | _____ Reps _____ Sets _____X Day _____Hold |
|---|---|
| **90** | **Notes:** |

SHOULDER ROLLS - WEIGHTS

Hold weights in both or one hand. Move your shoulders in a circular pattern  so that your are moving in an up, back and down direction.
Complete one set and then reverse direction

## Scapular Retraction

| | _____ Reps _____ Sets _____X Day _____Hold |
|---|---|
| **91** | **Notes:** |

SCAPULAR RETRACTIONS - BILATERAL

Draw your shoulder blades back and down.

| | _____ Reps _____ Sets _____X Day _____Hold |
|---|---|
| **92** | **Notes:** |

SCAPULAR RETRACTION – SINGLE ARM

With your arm raised up and elbow bent, draw your shoulder blade back and down.

| _____ Reps _____ Sets _____ X Day _____ Hold | | _____ Reps _____ Sets _____ X Day _____ Hold | |
|---|---|---|---|
| 93 | Notes: | 94 | Notes: |

ELASTIC BAND SCAPULAR RETRACTIONS WITH MINI SHOULDER EXTENSIONS

Fixate an elastic band to the door and hold with both arms in front of you with your elbows straight. Slowly squeeze your shoulder blades together as you pull the band back. Be sure your shoulders do not rise up.

PRONE RETRACTION – Can do without weight

Lie face down with your elbows straight. Slowly draw your shoulder blade back towards your spine. Your whole arm should rise including your shoulder blade upward as shown. Your elbow should be straight the entire time.

## Scapular Protraction

| _____ Reps _____ Sets _____ X Day _____ Hold | | _____ Reps _____ Sets _____ X Day _____ Hold | |
|---|---|---|---|
| 95 | Notes: | 96 | Notes: |

SCAPULAR PROTRACTION - SUPINE - BILATERAL

Lie on your back with your arms extended out in front of your body and towards the ceiling. While keeping your elbows straight, protract your shoulders reaching forward towards the ceiling. Keep your elbows straight the entire time.

SCAPULAR PROTRACTION - SUPINE - WEIGHT

Lie on your back holding a weight with your arm extended out in front of your body and towards the ceiling. While keeping your elbows straight, protract your shoulders reaching forward towards the ceiling. Keep your elbows straight the entire time.

| _____ Reps _____ Sets _____X Day _____Hold | _____ Reps _____ Sets _____X Day _____Hold |
|---|---|
| **97** Notes: | **98** Notes: |

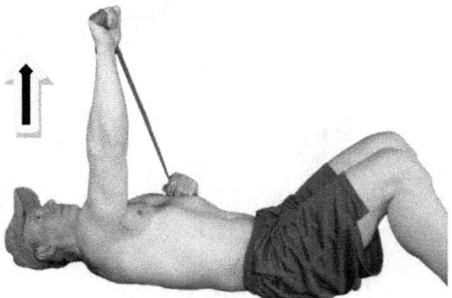

SCAPULAR PROTRACTION - SUPINE - ELASTIC BAND

Lie on your back and hold elastic band in both hands. Bend the unaffected arm to fixate the band. Extend the target arm out in front of your body and straight up towards the ceiling. While keeping your elbows straight, protract your shoulder blade forward towards the ceiling. Keep your elbows straight the entire time.

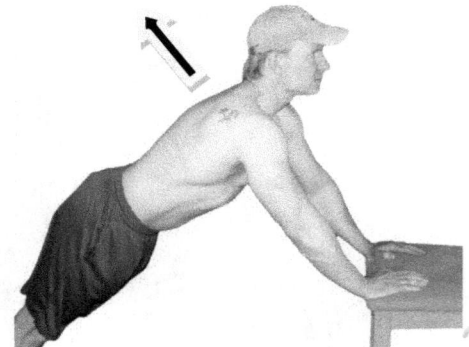

SCAPULAR PROTRACTION / TABLE PLANK

Start in a push up position on your hands and leaning up against a table or countertop as shown. Maintain this position as you protract your shoulder blades forward to raise your body upward a few inches. Return to original position.
*Progress by standing further away from the table.

## Chest Press

| _____ Reps _____ Sets _____X Day _____Hold | _____ Reps _____ Sets _____X Day _____Hold |
|---|---|
| **99** Notes: | **100** Notes: |

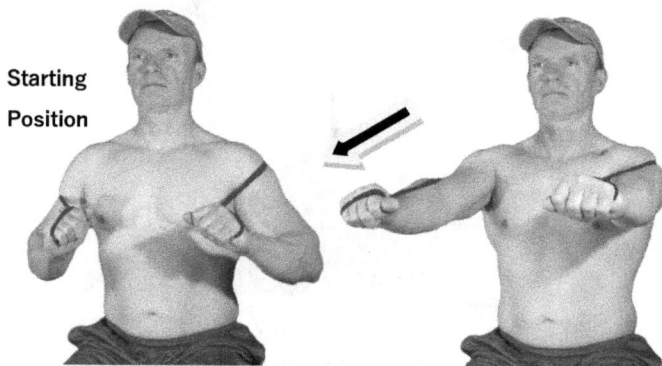

Starting Position

CHEST PRESS – SEATED or STANDING - ELASTIC BAND

Hold elastic band with both hands at your side and elbows bent with band wrapped around body or chair. Push the band out in front of your body as you straighten your elbows.

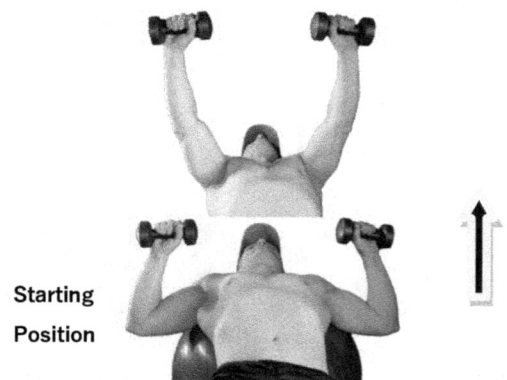

Starting Position

CHEST PRESS – BALL, FLOOR or BENCH- WEIGHTS

Lie on your back with your elbows bent. Slowly raise up your arms towards the ceiling while extending your elbows straight up above your head.

**Upper Extremity Strengthening**

| | _____ Reps _____ Sets _____X Day _____Hold |
|---|---|
| **101** | **Notes:** |

Starting
Position

DOWEL PRESS – STANDING – Add weight only if equal strength

Hold a dowel/cane at chest height. Slowly push the dowel outwards in front of your body so that your elbows become fully straightened. Return to the original position.

| | _____ Reps _____ Sets _____X Day _____Hold |
|---|---|
| **102** | **Notes:** |

Starting
Position

CHEST PRESS – STANDING or SEATED

Hold weights in both hands with your arms at your side and elbows bent. Push your arms out in front of your body as you straighten your elbows.

## Rows

| | _____ Reps _____ Sets _____X Day _____Hold |
|---|---|
| **103** | **Notes:** |

BENT OVER ROWS

Stand, bend over and support yourself with the unaffected arm. Slowly draw up your target arm as you bend your elbow. Keep your back flat the entire time.

| | _____ Reps _____ Sets _____X Day _____Hold |
|---|---|
| **104** | **Notes:** |

ROWS – PRONE – On bed or table

Lie face down with your elbows straight, slowly raise your arms upward while bending your elbows.

|  | _____ Reps _____ Sets _____ X Day _____ Hold |
|---|---|
| **105** | **Notes:** |

ROWS - ELASTIC BAND

Fixate the elastic band in the door at elbow level. Hold the elastic band with both hands, draw back the band as you bend your elbows. Keep your elbows near the side of your body.

|  | _____ Reps _____ Sets _____ X Day _____ Hold |
|---|---|
| **106** | **Notes:** |

WIDE ROWS - ELASTIC BAND

Fixate the elastic band in the door and hold the band with both hands. Draw back the band as you bend your elbows squeezing shoulder blades together. Keep your arms about 90 degrees away from the side of your body.

|  | _____ Reps _____ Sets _____ X Day _____ Hold |
|---|---|
| **107** | **Notes:** |

LOW ROW – ELASTIC BAND

Fixate the elastic band in the door below elbow level. Hold the elastic band with both hands, draw back the band as you bend your elbows. Keep your elbows near the side of your body.

|  | _____ Reps _____ Sets _____ X Day _____ Hold |
|---|---|
| **108** | **Notes:** |

HIGH ROW – ELASTIC BAND

Fixate the elastic band at the top of the door. Hold the elastic band with both hands, draw back the band as you bend your elbows. Keep your elbows near the side of your body.

## Flys

| | \_\_\_\_\_ Reps \_\_\_\_\_ Sets \_\_\_\_\_X Day \_\_\_\_\_Hold | | \_\_\_\_\_ Reps \_\_\_\_\_ Sets \_\_\_\_\_X Day \_\_\_\_\_Hold |
|---|---|---|---|
| **109** | **Notes:** | **110** | **Notes:** |

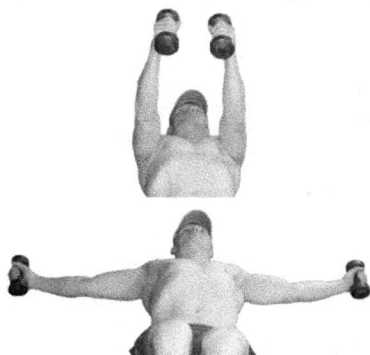

Starting

Position

FLY'S – FLOOR - WEIGHT

Holding weights, lie on your back with your arms horizontally out to the side. Bring your arms up and forward towards the ceiling. Lower your arms back down to the original position. Your elbows should be partially bent the entire time.

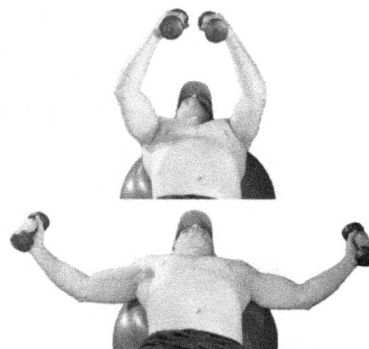

FLY'S – BALL or BENCH – WEIGHT

Holding weights, lie on your back on a ball with your arms horizontally out to the side. Bring your arms up and forward towards the ceiling. Lower your arms back down to the original position with elbows partially bent the entire time.

## Wall pushups – To progress, move feet further away from wall

| | \_\_\_\_\_ Reps \_\_\_\_\_ Sets \_\_\_\_\_X Day \_\_\_\_\_Hold | | \_\_\_\_\_ Reps \_\_\_\_\_ Sets \_\_\_\_\_X Day \_\_\_\_\_Hold |
|---|---|---|---|
| **111** | **Notes:** | **112** | **Notes:** |

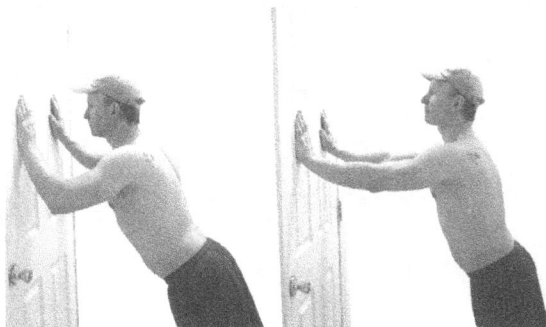

WALL PUSH UPS

Place your arms out in front of you with your elbows straight so that your hands just reach the wall. Bend your elbows slowly to bring your chest closer to the wall. Straighten your arms pushing your body away from wall. Maintain your feet planted on the ground the entire time.

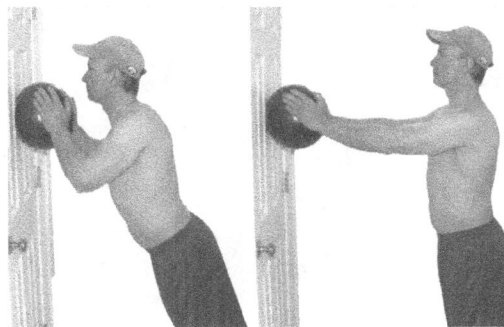

WALL PUSH UP - BALL

Place a ball on a wall while holding the ball with both hands as shown. Bend your elbows slowly to bring your chest closer to the wall and then straighten your arms pushing your body away from wall. Maintain your feet planted on the ground the entire time.

| | _____ Reps _____ Sets _____X Day _____Hold |
|---|---|
| **113** | **Notes:** |

WALL PUSH UP - Triceps uneven

Place your arms out in front of you with your elbows straight in an uneven position  so that your hands just reach the wall.  Bend your elbows slowly to bring your chest closer to the wall and then straighten your arms pushing your body away from wall. Maintain your feet planted on the ground the entire time.

| | _____ Reps _____ Sets _____X Day _____Hold |
|---|---|
| **114** | **Notes:** |

WALL PUSH UP – Hands inverted

Place your arms out in front of you with your elbows straight and hands inverted just reaching the wall.  Bend your elbows slowly to bring your chest closer to the wall and then straighten your arms pushing your body away from wall. Maintain your feet planted on the ground the entire time.

| | _____ Reps _____ Sets _____X Day _____Hold |
|---|---|
| **115** | **Notes:** |

WALL PUSH UP - Narrow

Place your arms out in front of you with your elbows straight and hands close togther just reaching the wall. Bend your elbows slowly to bring your chest closer to the wall and then straighten your arms pushing your body away from wall. Maintain your feet planted on the ground the entire time.

| | _____ Reps _____ Sets _____X Day _____Hold |
|---|---|
| **116** | **Notes:** |

WALL PUSH UP – Wide

Place your arms out in front of you with your elbows straight and your arms and  hands far apart just reaching the wall.  Bend your elbows slowly to bring your chest closer to the wall and then straighten your arms pushing your body away from wall. Maintain your feet planted on the ground the entire time.

# Push ups

| | _____ Reps _____ Sets _____ X Day _____ Hold | | _____ Reps _____ Sets _____ X Day _____ Hold |
|---|---|---|---|
| **117** | **Notes:** | **118** | **Notes:** |

Starting
Position

PUSH UPS - BALL

Start in a kneeling position with an exercise ball in front of you. Slowly walk yourself out with your arms so that the ball is positioned under your legs. Then perform push ups.
*Progress by moving ball back towards thighs

PUSH UP -  MODIFIED

Lie face down and use your arms and push yourself up.  Keep your knees in contact with the floor and maintain a straight back the entire time.

| | _____ Reps _____ Sets _____ X Day _____ Hold | | _____ Reps _____ Sets _____ X Day _____ Hold |
|---|---|---|---|
| **119** | **Notes:** | **120** | **Notes:** |

Starting
Position

PUSH UP

Lie face down, use your arms and push yourself.  Keep your toes in contact with the floor and maintain a straight back the entire time.

PUSH UP -DIAMOND

Lie face down and place your hands on the floor in the shape of a diamond with your thumbs and index fingers.
Use your arms and push yourself up..  Keep your toes in contact with the floor and maintain a straight back the entire time.

| | _____ Reps _____ Sets _____ X Day _____ Hold | | _____ Reps _____ Sets _____ X Day _____ Hold |
|---|---|---|---|
| **121** | **Notes:** | **122** | **Notes:** |

PUSH UP – MODIFIED - BOSU - UNSTABLE

Perform push-ups with your hands on a Bosu.  Keep your knees in contact with the floor and maintain a straight back the entire time.

PUSH UP – BOSU - UNSTABLE

Perform push-ups  with your hands on top of a Bosu.  Keep your toes in contact with the floor and maintain a straight back the entire time.

| | _____ Reps _____ Sets _____ X Day _____ Hold | | _____ Reps _____ Sets _____ X Day _____ Hold |
|---|---|---|---|
| **123** | **Notes:** | **124** | **Notes:** |

PUSH UP – MODIFIED – INVERTED BOSU - UNSTABLE

Perform push-ups while holding an inverted Bosu.  Try and maintain the Bosu platform as level as you can. Keep your knees in contact with the floor and maintain a straight back the entire time.

PUSH UP – INVERTED BOSU - UNSTABLE

Perform push-ups while holding an inverted Bosu. Try and maintain the Bosu platform as level as you can.  Keep your toes in contact with the floor and maintain a straight back the entire time.

# BALANCE – CORE – STANDING LE STRENGTH

Basics
- Requires LE strengthening for progression
- Perform exercises 2-3x a week
- Should be performed at beginning of exercise routine or can be the main exercise routine for endurance with increased repetitions or strength with resistance.

Duration, Frequency, Intensity, Sets and Reps
- Balance – 1 set, 2-4 repetitions for hold of 5-60 seconds
- Endurance – Less than 30 second rests in between sets
  - Static - 1 set, 5-10 repetitions as tolerated
  - Dynamic – 1 set, 3-10 reps for 10-30+ second hold as tolerated
- Strengthening – Add resistance with bands or weights (*see Strengthening for more information*)
  - Static – 2-3 sets, 3-12 reps – slow controlled movements
  - Dynamic – 1-3 sets, 2-4 reps

Static Balance Progression:
1. Bilateral – Both feet on the ground
2. Unilateral – One foot on the ground
3. Arm Movement – Overhead, can do arm exercises (*See Arm Strengthening for exercises*)
4. Trunk rotation – Rotate with or without arm movement
5. Eyes Shut (lack of visual cues – sensory removal)
6. Head Turns, hand/eye tracking, shifting focal point (vestibular – sensory alteration)
7. Reading (coordination)
8. Unstable – progression
   *Repeat above on unstable surface such as balance pad, pillow, balance disc or Bosu.*

Decrease Base of Support (BOS) Progression:
- Wide BOS
- Narrow Bos
- Staggered/Split Stance/Semi-tandem
- Tandem Stance
- Single Leg Stance

SOLID GROUND:
1. Support: Hold onto chair, counter, sink or another stationary object.
2. No Support: Stand next to stable surface if needed for security.
   - Can start with 1-2 hands and as you become more stable, decrease the number of fingers used for support. For example, take away the thumb and hold with 4 fingers, 3 fingers, 2 fingers, 1 finger and then without support.
3. Resistance: Add ankle weights on use elastic band for resistance

UNSTABLE SURFACE: Balance pad, Bosu, Half foam roll, Pillow or Other unstable surface
1. Support: Hold onto chair, counter or another stationary object.
2. No Support: Stand next to stable surface if needed for security.
   - Can start with 1-2 hands and as you become more stable, decrease the number of fingers used for support. For example, take away the thumb and hold with 4 fingers, 3 fingers, 2 fingers, 1 finger and then without support.
3. Resistance: Add ankle weights on use elastic band for resistance

| **Peripheral Neuropathy** <br><br> **Caution Balancing on Uneven Surface** | • Peripheral neuropathy can be a side effect of diabetes or may be as a result of damage to the peripheral nerves. These nerves carry information from the brain to other parts of the body. <br> • Feet or lower extremity – Caution standing on uneven surface, such as a Bosu ball or balance pads due to decreased sensation in feet. Increased risk of falling. <br> • Hands – Caution with holding dumbbells or grasping resistance bands. |
|---|---|

## Balance

| EXERCISE<br><br>Balance | EXERCISE NUMBER | NOTES |
|---|---|---|
| WIDE BOS DECREASING TO NARROW BOS | 1 | |
| NARROW BOS | 2 | |
| ARM MOVEMENT | 3 | |
| TRUNK ROTATION | 4 | |
| EYES SHUTS | 5 | |
| HEAD TURNS | 6 | |
| READING ALOUD | 7 | |
| BALANCE PAD | 8 | |
| SPLIT STANCE – SEMI TANDEM | 9 | |
| SPLIT STANCE - *Progression* | 10 | |
| TANDEM- SHARPENED ROMBERG STANCE | 11 | |
| TANDEM STANCE - Progression | 12 | |
| SINGLE LEG STANCE (SLS) | 13 | |
| SINGLE LEG STANCE (SLS) - *Progression* | 14 | |
| SLS – LEG FORWARD | 15 | |
| SLS – LEG BACKWARDS | 16 | |
| SLS – LEG FORWARD / OPPOSITE ARM UP | 17 | |
| SLS – LEG BACKWARDS / OPPOSITE ARM UP | 18 | |
| SLS - REACH FORWARD | 19 | |
| SLS - REACH TWIST | 20 | |
| SINGLE LEG TOE TAP | 21 | |
| SINGLE LEG STANCE - CLOCKS | 22 | |
| BALL ROLLS - HEEL TOE | 23 | |
| BALL ROLLS - LATERAL | 24 | |
| SQUAT | 25 | |
| SIT TO STAND | 26 | |

**Balance**

| EXERCISE Balance | EXERCISE NUMBER | NOTES |
|---|---|---|
| SQUATS – WALL WITH BALL | 27 | |
| SQUATS WITH WEIGHTS | 28 | |
| MINI SQUAT - UNSTABLE SUPPORT - FOAM PAD | 29 | |
| SQUATS - SINGLE LEG | 30 | |
| SIDE TO SIDE WEIGHT SHIFT | 31 | |
| FORWARD AND BACKWARDS WEIGHT SHIFTS | 32 | |
| SPLIT STANCE WEIGHT SHIFT SIDE TO SIDE | 33 | |
| SPLIT STANCE WEIGHT SHIFT FORWARD AND BACKWARDS | 34 | |
| WALL FALLS - FORWARD - BALANCE DRILL | 35 | |
| WALL FALLS - LATERAL - BALANCE DRILL | 36 | |
| WALL FALLS - BACKWARDS - BALANCE DRILL | 37 | |
| WALL FALLS - SINGLE LEG - FORWARD - BALANCE DRILL | 38 | |
| WALL FALLS - SINGLE LEG - LATERAL - BALANCE DRILL | 39 | |
| WALL FALLS - SINGLE LEG - MEDIAL - BALANCE DRILL | 40 | |
| WALL FALLS - SINGLE LEG - BACKWARDS - BALANCE DRILL | 41 | |
| FALL LATERAL - STEP RECOVERY | 42 | |
| FALL FORWARD - STEP RECOVERY | 43 | |
| FALL BACKWARD - STEP RECOVERY | 44 | |
| TOE TAP ABDUCTION | 45 | |
| HIP ABDUCTION - STANDING | 46 | |
| HIP EXTENSION – STANDING | 47 | |
| HIP FLEXION - STANDING – STRAIGHT LEG RAISE | 48 | |
| HIP / KNEE FLEXION - SINGLE LEG | 49 | |
| STANDING MARCHING | 50 | |

**Balance**

| EXERCISE<br><br>Balance | EXERCISE NUMBER | NOTES |
|---|---|---|
| HAMSTRING CURL | 51 | |
| TOE RAISES | 52 | |
| TOE RAISES IR AND ER | 53 | |
| ONE LEGGED TOE RAISE | 54 | |
| SINGLE LEG BALANCE FORWARD | 55 | |
| SINGLE LEG BALANCE LATERAL | 56 | |
| SINGLE LEG BALANCE RETRO | 57 | |
| SINGLE LEG STANCE RETROLATERAL | 58 | |
| SQUAT | 59 | |
| SINGLE LEG SQUAT | 60 | |
| LUNGE – STATIC | 61 | |
| LUNGE FORWARD/BACKWARD | 62 | |
| FOUR CORNER MARCHING IN PLACE | 63 | |
| FOUR CORNER MARCHING IN PLACE WITH HEAD TURNS | 64 | |
| WALKING ON HEELS FORWARD AND BACKWARDS | 65 | |
| WALKING ON TOES FORWARD AND BACKWARDS | 66 | |
| TANDEM STANCE AND WALK – FORWARD AND BACKWARDS | 67 | |
| RUNNING MAN | 68 | |
| HOP STICK - FORWARD | 69 | |
| HOP STICK - BACKWARDS | 70 | |
| MINI LATERAL LUNGE | 71 | |
| SIDE STEPPING | 72 | |
| HOP STICK - LATERAL | 73 | |
| SINGLE LEG DEAD LIFT | 74 | |

| EXERCISE<br><br>Balance | EXERCISE NUMBER | NOTES |
|---|---|---|
| CONE TAPS - SINGLE LEG STANCE | 75 | |
| CONE TAPS - SINGLE LEG STANCE - UNSTABLE | 76 | |
| FIGURE 8 AROUND CONES | 77 | |
| FIGURE 8 AROUND CONES – FOOT OR HAND TAP | 78 | |
| BALANCE DOUBLE LEG STANCE - WIDE | 79 | |
| BALANCE DOUBLE LEG STANCE - NARROW | 80 | |
| TANDEM STANCE | 81 | |
| TANDEM WALK | 82 | |
| SINGLE LEG STANCE - ABDUCTION | 83 | |
| SINGLE LEG STANCE - ABDUCTION | 84 | |
| SINGLE LEG STANCE – FORWARD KICK | 85 | |
| SINGLE LEG STANCE – HAMSTRING CURL | 86 | |
| SINGLE LEG SQUAT – LEG FORWARD | 87 | |
| SINGLE LEG SQUAT – LEG BACKWARDS | 88 | |
| TOE TAP OR HEEL PLACEMENT | 89 | |
| PULL UP FOOT TOUCHES ON STEP | 90 | |
| ALTERNATING SUSTAINED FOOT TOUCHES ON STEP | 91 | |
| STEP UP AND OVER | 92 | |
| FORWARD SWING THROUGH STEP | 93 | |
| SIDE STEPPING - *REPEAT STEPS 89-93 from a side approach.* | 94 | |

## BALANCE PROGRESSION- STATIC – See WARNING above Re: Peripheral Neuropathy

**Hip Width/Narrow Stance  >>>>>   Staggered Stance  >>>>>  Tandem Stance      >>>>>  Single-Leg Stance**

1. Hold onto a chair, counter or other steady object.
2. Continue steps 2-8 holding on to a sturdy object.
3. Can start with 1-2 hands and as you become more stable, decrease the number of fingers used for support.  For example, take away the thumb and hold with 4 fingers, 3 fingers, 2 fingers, 1 finger and then without support.
4. When feeling comfortable, take away support staying close to object for security
5. When able to complete with decreased support, add balance pad or unstable surface completing 2-8 as above.

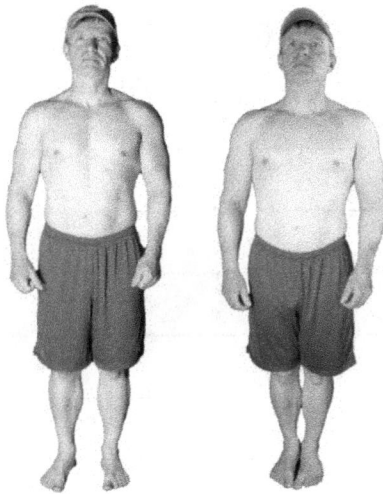

HIP WIDTH OR WIDE BASE OF SUPPORT (BOS) > NARROW BASE OF SUPPORT (BOS)

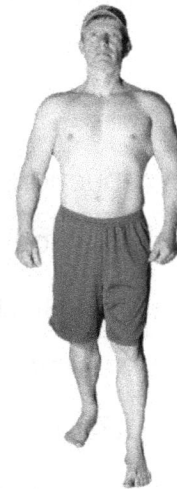

STAGGERED STANCE – SPLIT STANCE

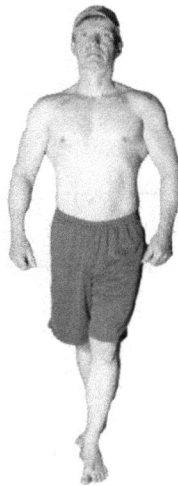

TANDEM STANCE

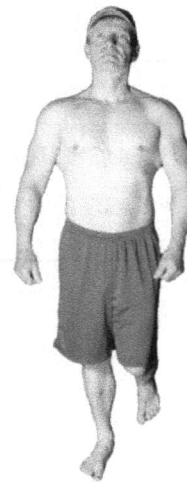

SINGLE LEG STANCE

**Balance**

| | _____ Reps _____ Sets _____ X Day _____ Hold | | _____ Reps _____ Sets _____ X Day _____ Hold |
|---|---|---|---|
| **1** | **Notes:** | **2** | **Notes:** |

WIDE BOS DECREASING TO NARROW BOS

_Continue steps 2-8 holding on to a sturdy object and then progress with decreased support as outlined above._

NARROW BOS

Stand with your feet together Count to 10. Increase time up to 60 seconds as tolerated maintaining your balance in this position.

| | _____ Reps _____ Sets _____ X Day _____ Hold | | _____ Reps _____ Sets _____ X Day _____ Hold |
|---|---|---|---|
| **3** | **Notes:** | **4** | **Notes:** |

ARM MOVEMENT

Examples:
- Throw ball up in arm and catch
- Play catch with partner
- Reach hands above head and then down by side
- Do standing arm exercises (_See Arm Strengthening for examples_)

TRUNK ROTATION – reach side to side

Examples:
- Reach side to side within BOS
- Reach side to side and forward out of BOS

| | \_\_\_\_\_ Reps \_\_\_\_\_ Sets \_\_\_\_\_ X Day \_\_\_\_\_ Hold | | | \_\_\_\_\_ Reps \_\_\_\_\_ Sets \_\_\_\_\_ X Day \_\_\_\_\_ Hold |
|---|---|---|---|---|
| **5** | **Notes:** | | **6** | **Notes:** |

EYES SHUTS - Lack of visual cues – *Sensory Removal*

Stand with eyes shut and count to 10.  Increase time up to 60 seconds as tolerated.

HEAD TURNS - Vestibular – *Sensory Alteration*

Examples:
- Turn head slowly from side to side
- Move head up and down slowly
- Put one finger out in front of face at arm's length moving in outward/inward direction and move head to follow with eyes. Slow hand tracking.
- Shift focal point to different objects in the room
- *Can add head turns with eyes closed*

| | \_\_\_\_\_ Reps \_\_\_\_\_ Sets \_\_\_\_\_ X Day \_\_\_\_\_ Hold | | | \_\_\_\_\_ Reps \_\_\_\_\_ Sets \_\_\_\_\_ X Day \_\_\_\_\_ Hold |
|---|---|---|---|---|
| **7** | **Notes:** | | **8** | **Notes:** |

READING ALOUD - *Coordination / Cognitive Task*

Hold reading material, such as a book, paper, tablet, or magazine in one or both hands.  Read out loud and progress to moving your head and the object on occasion to the side or up/down.

BALANCE PAD or another unstable surface

Place balance pad, Bosu, pillow or other unstable surface by a chair or counter for support. Stand on the pad.

**\*\*\*\*REPEAT STEPS 2-8 on unstable surface\*\*\*\***

| | | |
|---|---|---|
| | _____ Reps _____ Sets _____ X Day _____ Hold | _____ Reps _____ Sets _____ X Day _____ Hold |
| **9** | **Notes:** | **10** **Notes:** |

SPLIT STANCE – SEMI TANDEM

Place one foot forward and the opposite foot to the back and slightly out to the side. Count to 10. Increase time up to 60 seconds as tolerated maintaining your balance in this position.

**SPLIT STANCE**

**_FOLLOW STEPS 2-8 AS SEEN WITH NARROW BOS AS OUTLINED IN BALANCE PROGRESSION_**

1. HOLD STEADY OBJECT PROGRESSING TO NO SUPPORT
2. STAND FOR 10-60 SECONDS
3. ARM MOVEMENT
4. TRUNK ROTATION
5. EYES SHUT
6. HEAD TURNS
7. READING
8. **UNSTABLE**

REPEAT ABOVE ON UNSTABLE SURFACE SUCH AS BALANCE PAD, PILLOW, BALANCE DISC, HALF FOARM ROLL OR BOSU.

| | | |
|---|---|---|
| | _____ Reps _____ Sets _____ X Day _____ Hold | _____ Reps _____ Sets _____ X Day _____ Hold |
| **11** | **Notes:** | **12** **Notes:** |

TANDEM- SHARPENED ROMBERG STANCE

Place the heel of one foot so that it touches the toes of the other foot. Count to 10. Increase time up to 60 seconds as tolerated maintaining your balance in this position.

**TANDEM STANCE**

**_FOLLOW STEPS 2-8 AS SEEN WITH NARROW BOS AS OUTLINED IN BALANCE PROGRESSION_**

1. HOLD STEADY OBJECT PROGRESSING TO NO SUPPORT
2. STAND FOR 10-60 SECONDS
3. ARM MOVEMENT
4. TRUNK ROTATION
5. EYES SHUT
6. HEAD TURNS
7. READING
8. **UNSTABLE**

REPEAT ABOVE ON UNSTABLE SURFACE SUCH AS BALANCE PAD, PILLOW, BALANCE DISC, HALF FOARM ROLL OR BOSU.

| | _____ Reps _____ Sets _____X Day _____Hold | | _____ Reps _____ Sets _____X Day _____Hold |
|---|---|---|---|
| **13** | Notes: | **14** | Notes: |

SINGLE LEG STANCE (SLS)

Stand on one foot. Count to 10 > 60 seconds as tolerated maintaining your balance in this position. Maintain a slightly bent knee on the stance side.

### SINGLE LEG STANCE

***FOLLOW STEPS 2-8 AS SEEN WITH NARROW BOS AS OUTLINED IN BALANCE PROGRESSION***

1. HOLD STEADY OBJECT PROGRESSING TO NO SUPPORT
2. STAND FOR 10-60 SECONDS
3. ARM MOVEMENT
4. TRUNK ROTATION
5. EYES SHUT
6. HEAD TURNS
7. READING
8. **UNSTABLE**

REPEAT ABOVE ON UNSTABLE SURFACE SUCH AS BALANCE PAD, PILLOW, BALANCE DISC, HALF FOARM ROLL OR BOSU.

## Single Leg Stance (SLS) with Arm and/or Leg Movements- *Progress to Balance Pad*

| | _____ Reps _____ Sets _____X Day _____Hold | | _____ Reps _____ Sets _____X Day _____Hold |
|---|---|---|---|
| **15** | Notes: | **16** | Notes: |

SLS – LEG FORWARD

Stand on one leg and maintain your balance. Hold your leg out in front of your body and then return to the original position. Repeat on opposite side. Maintain a slightly bent knee on the stance side.

SLS – LEG BACKWARDS

Stand on one leg and maintain your balance. Hold your leg in the back of your body and then return to original position. Repeat on opposite side. Maintain a slightly bent knee on the stance side.

| _____ Reps _____ Sets _____ X Day _____ Hold | | _____ Reps _____ Sets _____ X Day _____ Hold |
|---|---|---|
| **17** | Notes: | **18** Notes: |

**SLS – LEG FORWARD / OPPOSITE ARM UP**

Stand on one leg and maintain your balance. Hold your leg out in front of your body and opposite arm up over your head.  Return to the original position. Repeat on opposite side.  Maintain a slightly bent knee on the stance side.

**SLS – LEG BACKWARDS / OPPOSITE ARM UP**

Stand on one leg and maintain your balance. Hold your leg out in front of your body and opposite arm up over your head.  Return to the original position. Repeat on opposite side.  Maintain a slightly bent knee on the stance side.

| _____ Reps _____ Sets _____ X Day _____ Hold | | _____ Reps _____ Sets _____ X Day _____ Hold |
|---|---|---|
| **19** | Notes: | **20** Notes: |

**SLS - REACH FORWARD**

Stand on one leg and maintain your balance.  Reach forward with your opposite arm as far as you can without losing your balance and then return to original position. Repeat on opposite side.  Maintain a slightly bent knee on the stance side.

**SLS - REACH TWIST**

Stand on one leg and maintain your balance. Reach forward and across your body with your opposite arm as far as you can without losing your balance and then return to original position. Repeat on opposite side.  Maintain a slightly bent knee on the stance side.

| | _____ Reps _____ Sets _____X Day _____Hold | | _____ Reps _____ Sets _____X Day _____Hold |
|---|---|---|---|
| **21** | **Notes:** | **22** | **Notes:** |

SINGLE LEG TOE TAP

Start by standing on one leg and maintain your balance. Tap the opposite foot on a slightly raised object, such as a box or balance pad.  To progress, increase the height of object, such as a stair step or cone.  Can alternate feet or repeat on same side for several repetitions and then repeat on opposite side.

SINGLE LEG STANCE - CLOCKS

Start by standing on one leg and maintain your balance. Image a clock on the floor where your stance leg is in the center.  Lightly touch position 1 as illustrated with the opposite foot. Then return that leg to the starting position.  Next, touch position 2 and return. Maintain a slightly bent knee on the stance side.

| | _____ Reps _____ Sets _____X Day _____Hold | | _____ Reps _____ Sets _____X Day _____Hold |
|---|---|---|---|
| **23** | **Notes:** | **24** | **Notes:** |

BALL ROLLS - HEEL TOE

In a standing position, place one foot on a ball and roll it forward and back in a controlled motion from heel to toe while maintaining your balance.

BALL ROLLS - LATERAL

In a standing position, place one foot on a ball and roll it side to side in a controlled motion from the inner side of your foot to the outer side of your foot while maintaining your balance.

## Squats

| | |
|---|---|
| _____ Reps _____ Sets _____ X Day _____ Hold | _____ Reps _____ Sets _____ X Day _____ Hold |
| **25** Notes: | **26** Notes: |

SQUAT – Can use chair or counter for support and chair behind if needed.

Stand with feet shoulder width apart (in front of a stable support for balance if needed.) Bend your knees and lower your body towards the floor. Your body weight should mostly be directed through the heels of your feet. Return to a standing position. Knees should bend in line with toes and not pass the front of the foot.

SIT TO STAND - Can use armchair to push off if needed

Start by scooting close to the front of the chair. Lean forward at your trunk and reach forward with your arms and rise to standing. (You may use a chair with arms to push off if needed and progress as tolerated).
Use your arms as a counterbalance by reaching forward when in sitting and lower them as you approach standing.

| | |
|---|---|
| _____ Reps _____ Sets _____ X Day _____ Hold | _____ Reps _____ Sets _____ X Day _____ Hold |
| **27** Notes: | **28** Notes: |

SQUATS – WALL WITH BALL

Place either a small ball or therapy ball between you and the wall. Bend your knees and lower your body towards the floor. Return to a standing position. Knees should bend in line with toes and not pass the front of the foot.

SQUATS WITH WEIGHTS

Hold dumbbells or other weights in both hands by your side. Bend your knees and lower your body towards the floor. Return to a standing position. Knees should bend in line with toes and not pass the front of the foot

| | _____ Reps _____ Sets _____ X Day _____ Hold |
|---|---|
| **29** | **Notes:** |

MINI SQUAT - UNSTABLE SUPPORT - FOAM PAD

Start with your feet shoulder-width apart, toes pointed straight ahead and standing on a balance pad. Next, bend your knees to approximately 30 degrees of flexion to perform a mini squat as shown. Then, return to original position. Knees should not pass the front of the foot.

| | _____ Reps _____ Sets _____ X Day _____ Hold |
|---|---|
| **30** | **Notes:** |

SQUATS - SINGLE LEG

While standing on one leg in front of a stable support for assisted balance, bend your knee and lower your body towards the floor. Return to a standing position.
Knees should not pass the front of the foot.

## Weight Shifts, Wall Falls, Balance Recovery (Balance Drills)

| | _____ Reps _____ Sets _____ X Day _____ Hold |
|---|---|
| **31** | **Notes:** |

SIDE TO SIDE WEIGHT SHIFT
Stand next to stable surface if needed for support.

Keep feet shoulder width apart. Lean from side to side maintaining balance. *May stand in hallway with walls on both sides.*
*Advance to using balance pad

| | _____ Reps _____ Sets _____ X Day _____ Hold |
|---|---|
| **32** | **Notes:** |

FORWARD AND BACKWARDS WEIGHT SHIFTS
Stand next to stable surface if needed for support.

Keep feet shoulder width apart. Lean from body forward and then backwards maintaining balance. *May stand in hallway with wall in front and in back.*
 *Advance to using balance pad

| | _____ Reps _____ Sets _____ X Day _____ Hold |
|---|---|
| **33** | **Notes:** |

SPLIT STANCE WEIGHT SHIFT SIDE TO SIDE
Stand next to stable surface if needed for support.

Stand in a split stance position. Lean side to side maintaining balance. _May stand in hallway with wall on both sides._

| | _____ Reps _____ Sets _____ X Day _____ Hold |
|---|---|
| **34** | **Notes:** |

SPLIT STANCE WEIGHT SHIFT FORWARD AND BACKWARDS Stand next to stable surface if needed for support.

Stand in a split stance position. Lean forward and backwards maintaining balance. _May stand in hallway with wall in front and in back._

| | _____ Reps _____ Sets _____ X Day _____ Hold |
|---|---|
| **35** | **Notes:** |

WALL FALLS - FORWARD - BALANCE DRILL

Stand facing wall, a couple feet away from the wall. Slowly and controlled, lean forward towards the wall. Try to control your balance to prevent falling forward. Keep leaning forward gradually until eventually you do lose your balance and fall. Use your arms to catch yourself. Push yourself back upright.

| | _____ Reps _____ Sets _____ X Day _____ Hold |
|---|---|
| **36** | **Notes:** |

WALL FALLS - LATERAL - BALANCE DRILL

Stand to the side next to a wall, a couple feet away from the wall. Slowly and controlled, lean to the side towards the wall. Try to control your balance to prevent falling sideways. Keep leaning to the side gradually until eventually you do lose your balance and fall. Use your arm to catch yourself. Push yourself back upright.

| | _____ Reps _____ Sets _____ X Day _____ Hold | | _____ Reps _____ Sets _____ X Day _____ Hold |
|---|---|---|---|
| **37** | **Notes:** | **38** | **Notes:** |

**WALL FALLS - BACKWARDS - BALANCE DRILL**

Stand facing away from a wall. Slowly and controlled, lean backward towards the wall. Try to control your balance to prevent falling backwards. Keep leaning backwards gradually until eventually you do lose your balance and fall. Use your upper back to catch the fall. Push yourself back upright.

**WALL FALLS - SINGLE LEG - FORWARD - BALANCE DRILL**

Stand on one leg facing a wall, a couple feet away from the wall. Slowly and controlled, lean forward towards the wall. Try to control your balance to prevent falling forward. Keep leaning forward gradually until eventually you do lose your balance and fall. Use your arms to catch yourself. Push yourself back upright.

| | _____ Reps _____ Sets _____ X Day _____ Hold | | _____ Reps _____ Sets _____ X Day _____ Hold |
|---|---|---|---|
| **39** | **Notes:** | **40** | **Notes:** |

**WALL FALLS - SINGLE LEG - LATERAL - BALANCE DRILL**

Stand on one leg with a wall a couple feet off to the side of that leg. Slowly and controlled, lean to the side towards the wall. Try to control your balance to prevent falling to the side. Keep leaning gradually towards the wall until eventually you lose your balance and fall. Use your arms to catch yourself. Push yourself back upright.

**WALL FALLS - SINGLE LEG - MEDIAL - BALANCE DRILL**

Stand on one leg with a wall a couple feet off to the opposite side of that leg as shown. Slowly and controlled, lean sideways towards the wall. Try to control your balance to prevent falling to the side. Keep leaning gradually towards the wall until eventually you lose your balance and fall. Use your arms to catch yourself. Push yourself back upright.

| _____ Reps _____ Sets _____ X Day _____ Hold | | _____ Reps _____ Sets _____ X Day _____ Hold |
|---|---|---|
| **41** | Notes: | **42** | Notes: |

**WALL FALLS - SINGLE LEG - BACKWARDS - BALANCE DRILL**

Stand on one leg facing away from a wall. Slowly and controlled, lean backward towards the wall. Try and control your balance to prevent falling backwards. Keep leaning backwards gradually until eventually you do lose your balance and fall. Use your upper back to catch the fall. Push yourself back upright.

**FALL LATERAL - STEP RECOVERY**
Stand next to stable surface if needed for support.

Start in a standing position with feet apart. Slowly lean to the side and try and prevent losing your balance. Continue to lean to the side until eventually you lose your balance and need to take a step to prevent falling.

| _____ Reps _____ Sets _____ X Day _____ Hold | | _____ Reps _____ Sets _____ X Day _____ Hold |
|---|---|---|
| **43** | Notes: | **44** | Notes: |

**FALL FORWARD - STEP RECOVERY**
Stand next to stable surface if needed for support.

Start in a standing position with feet apart. Slowly lean forward and try and prevent losing your balance. Continue to lean forward until eventually you lose your balance and need to take a step to prevent falling.

**FALL BACKWARD - STEP RECOVERY**
Stand next to stable surface if needed for support.

Start in a standing position with feet apart. Slowly lean back and try and prevent losing your balance. Continue to lean backwards until eventually you lose your balance and need to take a step to prevent falling.

## LEG EXERCISES > BALANCE > RESISTANCE

**SOLID GROUND:**
1. **Support:** Hold onto chair, counter, sink or another stationary object
2. **No Support:** Stand next to stable surface if needed for support
3. **Resistance:** Add ankle weights on use elastic band for resistance

**UNSTABLE SURFACE:** Balance pad, Bosu, Half foam roll, Pillow or Other unstable surface
1. **Support:** Hold onto chair, counter or another stationary object.
2. **No Support:** Stand next to stable surface if needed for support.
3. **Resistance:** Add ankle weights on use elastic band for resistance

*Peripheral Neuropathy* – See beginning of section for Caution on Unstable Surface

| | _____ Reps _____ Sets _____X Day _____Hold | | _____ Reps _____ Sets _____X Day _____Hold |
|---|---|---|---|
| 45 | Notes: | 46 | Notes: |

TOE TAP ABDUCTION

Standing upright and move your leg out to the side and tap your toe on the ground. Return to starting position and repeat.

HIP ABDUCTION - STANDING – Can add ankle weights or elastic band.

Standing upright, raise your leg out to the side. Keep your knee straight and maintain your toes pointed forward the entire time. Return to starting position and repeat. Maintain a slow, controlled movement throughout.

**Balance**

| | _____ Reps _____ Sets _____ X Day _____ Hold | | _____ Reps _____ Sets _____ X Day _____ Hold |
|---|---|---|---|
| 47 | Notes: | 48 | Notes: |

HIP EXTENSION – STANDING - Can add ankle weights or band.

Standing upright, balance on one leg and move your other leg in a backward direction. Do not swing the leg and tighten the buttock at end range. Keep your trunk stable and without arching or bending forward during the movement. Return to starting position and repeat. Maintain a slow, controlled movement throughout.

HIP FLEXION - STANDING – STRAIGHT LEG RAISE - Can add ankle weights or band.

Standing upright, balance on one leg and lift your other leg forward with a straight knee as shown. Return to starting position and repeat. Maintain a slow, controlled movement throughout.

| | _____ Reps _____ Sets _____ X Day _____ Hold | | _____ Reps _____ Sets _____ X Day _____ Hold |
|---|---|---|---|
| 49 | Notes: | 50 | Notes: |

HIP / KNEE FLEXION - SINGLE LEG - Can add ankle weights

Standing upright, lift your foot and knee up, set it down. Repeat. Maintain a slow, controlled movement throughout.

STANDING MARCHING- Can add ankle weights

Standing upright, draw up your knee, set it down and then alternate to your other side. Maintain a slow, controlled movement throughout.

| | _____ Reps _____ Sets _____ X Day _____ Hold |
|---|---|
| **51** | **Notes:** |

HAMSTRING CURL - Can add ankle weights.

Standing upright, balance on one leg while bending the knee of the opposite leg towards the buttocks. Return to starting position and repeat.  Maintain a slow, controlled movement throughout.

| | _____ Reps _____ Sets _____ X Day _____ Hold |
|---|---|
| **52** | **Notes:** |

TOE RAISES - Can add hand weights.

Standing upright, go up on your toes slowly towards the ceiling and then return to the starting position. Maintain a slow, controlled movement throughout.

| | _____ Reps _____ Sets _____ X Day _____ Hold |
|---|---|
| **53** | **Notes:** |

TOE RAISES IR AND ER - Can add hand weights.

**IR** (Internal Rotation)
Standing upright, rotate feet/legs inward and go up on your toes slowly towards the ceiling and then return to the starting position.  Maintain a slow, controlled movement throughout.
**ER** (External Rotation)
Standing upright, rotate feet/legs outward and go up on your toes slowly towards the ceiling and then return to the starting position.

| | _____ Reps _____ Sets _____ X Day _____ Hold |
|---|---|
| **54** | **Notes:** |

ONE LEGGED TOE RAISE - Can add hand weights.

Standing upright and balance on one leg.  Go up on your toes on the opposite leg towards the ceiling and then return to the starting position. Maintain a slow, controlled movement throughout.

# BOSU – Can use chair for stability

| _____ Reps _____ Sets _____X Day _____Hold | | _____ Reps _____ Sets _____X Day _____Hold |
|---|---|---|

**55** Notes:

**56** Notes:

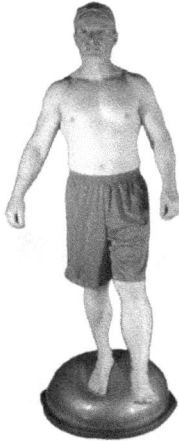

**SINGLE LEG BALANCE FORWARD**

Stand on a Bosu with one leg and maintain your balance. Hold your opposite leg out in front of your body and then return to original position. Maintain a slightly bent knee on the stance side.

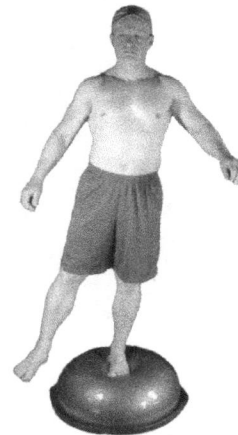

**SINGLE LEG BALANCE LATERAL**

Stand on a Bosu with one leg and maintain your balance. Hold your opposite leg out to the side of your body and then return to original position. Maintain a slightly bent knee on the stance side.

| _____ Reps _____ Sets _____X Day _____Hold | | _____ Reps _____ Sets _____X Day _____Hold |
|---|---|---|

**57** Notes:

**58** Notes:

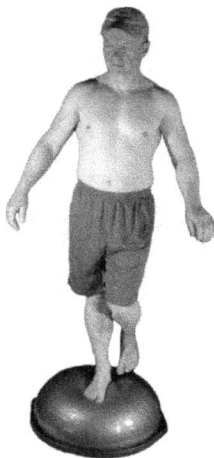

**SINGLE LEG BALANCE RETRO**

Stand on a Bosu Ball with one leg and maintain your balance. Hold your opposite leg back behind your body and then return to original position. Maintain a slightly bent knee on the stance side.

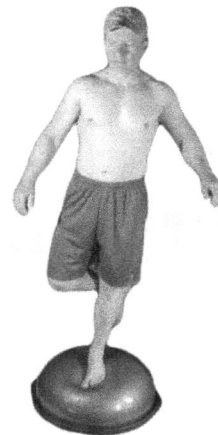

**SINGLE LEG STANCE RETROLATERAL**

Stand on a Bosu Ball with one leg and maintain your balance. Hold your opposite leg back behind and across your body and then return to original position. Maintain a slightly bent knee on the stance side.

| | _____ Reps _____ Sets _____X Day _____Hold |
|---|---|
| **59** | **Notes:** |

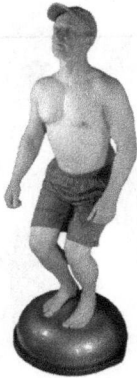

SQUAT

While standing and maintaining your balance on a Bosu, squat and return to a standing position. Knees should bend in line with the 2nd toe and not pass the front of the foot.

| | _____ Reps _____ Sets _____X Day _____Hold |
|---|---|
| **60** | **Notes:** |

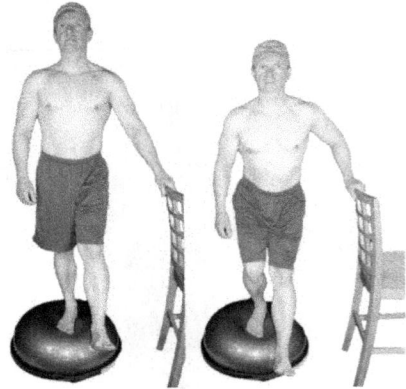

SINGLE LEG SQUAT

While standing and balancing on a Bosu with one leg, bend your knee and lower your body towards the ground. Return to a standing position. Your stance knee should bend in line with the 2nd toe and not pass the front of the foot.

## Lunges

| | _____ Reps _____ Sets _____X Day _____Hold |
|---|---|
| **61** | **Notes:** |

Starting Position

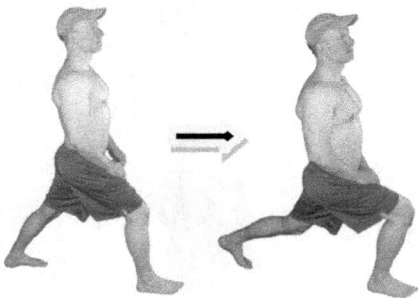

LUNGE – STATIC

Start in standing position with back leg straight and front leg with flexed/bent knee. Lean forward on front knee keeping knee in line with foot and back leg remaining straight. Return to starting position and repeat for several repetitions and then repeat on opposite side. *Make sure front knee does not go past the foot.

| | _____ Reps _____ Sets _____X Day _____Hold |
|---|---|
| **62** | **Notes:** |

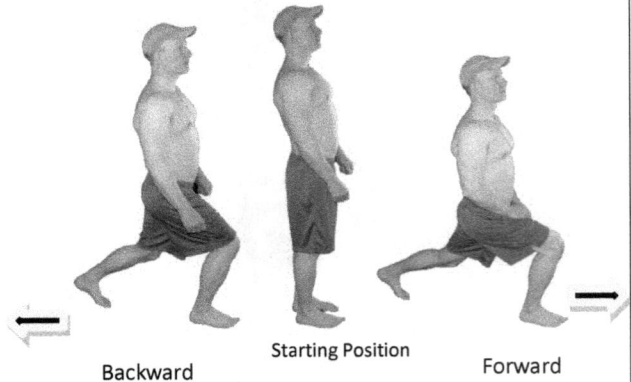

Backward          Starting Position          Forward

LUNGE FORWARD/BACKWARD

Start in standing (_middle picture_).
_Backward:_ Keep one foot planted and step back with the opposite foot. Return to original position - repeat. _Forward:_ Keep one foot planted and step forward with the opposite foot. Return to original position - repeat.

## DYNAMIC MOVEMENTS

| | | | |
|---|---|---|---|
| | _____ Reps _____ Sets _____ X Day _____ Hold | | _____ Reps _____ Sets _____ X Day _____ Hold |
| **63** | Notes: | **64** | Notes: |

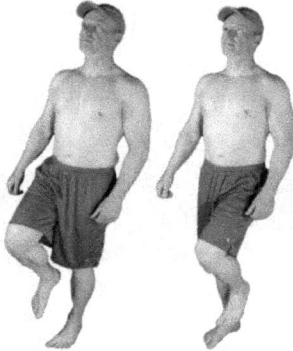

**FOUR CORNER MARCHING IN PLACE**

Marching in place, move your body clockwise stopping at each corner for several seconds and move to the next corner. After completing the square, march counterclockwise.

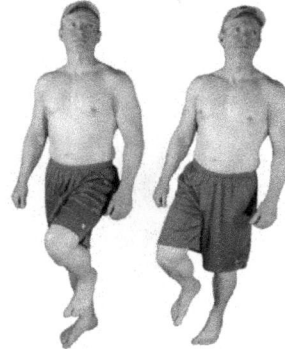

**FOUR CORNER MARCHING IN PLACE WITH HEAD TURNS**

*With Head and Body Moving Simultaneously*
March in place to four corners, as previous exercise (#63). Move your head and body moving simultaneously as you complete the square.
*With Head Turn And Then Body Turn.*
March in place to four corners, as previous exercise (#63). Turn head and then body as you complete the square.

| | | | |
|---|---|---|---|
| | _____ Reps _____ Sets _____ X Day _____ Hold | | _____ Reps _____ Sets _____ X Day _____ Hold |
| **65** | Notes: | **66** | Notes: |

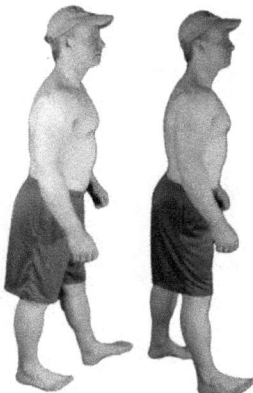

**WALKING ON HEELS FORWARD AND BACKWARDS** – May walk along kitchen counter or wall until feeling steady.

Standing up tall, walk forward on heels. After feeling secure with a forward motion, try walking backwards on heels.

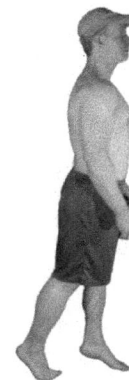

**WALKING ON TOES FORWARD AND BACKWARDS** – May walk along kitchen counter or wall until feeling steady.

Standing up tall, walk forward on up on toes. After feeling secure with a forward motion, try walking backwards up on toes.

| | _____ Reps _____ Sets _____X Day _____Hold |
|---|---|
| **67** | **Notes:** |

TANDEM STANCE AND WALK – FORWARD AND BACKWARDS

Maintaining your balance, stand with one foot directly in front of the other so that the toes of one foot touches the heel of the other. Progress by taking steps with your heel touching your toes with each step.
**Progress by walking backwards with your toe touching your heel with each step. Can also add head turns.

| | _____ Reps _____ Sets _____X Day _____Hold |
|---|---|
| **68** | **Notes:** |

RUNNING MAN

Stand and balance on one leg. Lean forward as you bring your other leg back behind you to tap the floor. Bring the same side arm forward as shown during the movement. Return to starting position and repeat.

| | _____ Reps _____ Sets _____X Day _____Hold |
|---|---|
| **69** | **Notes:** |

HOP STICK - FORWARD

Stand on one leg and then hop forward onto the other leg. Maintain your balance the entire time. Increase the difficulty by hoping forward further or higher.

| | _____ Reps _____ Sets _____X Day _____Hold |
|---|---|
| **70** | **Notes:** |

HOP STICK - BACKWARDS

Stand on one leg and then hop backward onto the other leg. Maintain your balance the entire time. Increase the difficulty by hoping back further or higher.

| | _____ Reps _____ Sets _____ X Day _____ Hold |
|---|---|
| **71** | **Notes:** |

MINI LATERAL LUNGE

Step to the side and balance on the leg. Next return to the original position. Repeat in the opposite direction. Your knees should be bent about 30 degrees.

| | _____ Reps _____ Sets _____ X Day _____ Hold |
|---|---|
| **72** | **Notes:** |

SIDE STEPPING – May step along kitchen counter or in hallway for support.

Step to the side continuing for length of room or counter – repeat in opposite direction.

| | _____ Reps _____ Sets _____ X Day _____ Hold |
|---|---|
| **73** | **Notes:** |

HOP STICK - LATERAL

Stand on one leg and then hop to the side onto the other leg. Maintain your balance the entire time. Increase the difficulty by hoping to the side further and higher.

| | _____ Reps _____ Sets _____ X Day _____ Hold |
|---|---|
| **74** | **Notes:** |

SINGLE LEG DEAD LIFT

While standing on one leg, bend forward with arms in front towards the ground as you extend your leg behind you and then return to the original position. Keep your legs straight and maintain your balance the entire time.

**Balance**

| | _____ Reps _____ Sets _____X Day _____Hold |
|---|---|
| **75** | **Notes:** |

CONE TAPS - SINGLE LEG STANCE

Place 3-5 cones or cups around you as shown. Balance on a slightly bent knee. Lower yourself down to tap the top of a cone with your finger. Return to original position and repeat touching a different cone. Advance exercise with smaller cones/cups and or faster speed.

| | _____ Reps _____ Sets _____X Day _____Hold |
|---|---|
| **76** | **Notes:** |

CONE TAPS - SINGLE LEG STANCE - UNSTABLE

Place 3-5 cones or cups around you. Balance on an unstable surface such as a foam pad with a slightly bent knee. Lower yourself down to tap the top of a cone. Return to original position and repeat touching a different cone. Advance exercise with smaller cones/cups and or faster speed.

| | _____ Reps _____ Sets _____X Day _____Hold |
|---|---|
| **77** | **Notes:** |

FIGURE 8 AROUND CONES

Set up 4-8 cones on the floor about 12 inches apart, although can vary to increase or decrease difficulty. Weave in and out of cones and then turn and repeat.

| | _____ Reps _____ Sets _____X Day _____Hold |
|---|---|
| **78** | **Notes:** |

FIGURE 8 AROUND CONES – FOOT OR HAND TAP

Follow #75 figure around 4- 8 cones. To increase difficulty, you can tap each cone with your foot or lean over and tap with your hand.

## HALF ROLLER (static and dynamic) – FLAT SIDE UP OR DOWN

| | _____ Reps _____ Sets _____ X Day _____ Hold | | _____ Reps _____ Sets _____ X Day _____ Hold |
|---|---|---|---|
| **79** | Notes: | **80** | Notes: |

**BALANCE DOUBLE LEG STANCE - WIDE**

Place a half foam roll on the ground in a side-to-side direction. Stand on the foam roll with your feet spread apart and maintain your balance.

**BALANCE DOUBLE LEG STANCE - NARROW**

Place a half foam roll on the ground in a side-to-side direction. Stand on the foam roll with your feet together and maintain your balance.

| | _____ Reps _____ Sets _____ X Day _____ Hold | | _____ Reps _____ Sets _____ X Day _____ Hold |
|---|---|---|---|
| **81** | Notes: | **82** | Notes: |

**TANDEM STANCE**

Place a half foam roll on the ground in a forward-back direction. Stand on the foam roll in tandem stance (with your heel and toe touching as shown) and maintain your balance.

**TANDEM WALK**

Place a half foam roll on the ground in a forward-back direction. Stand on the foam roll and begin tandem walking (heel-toe pattern walking as shown). Once you get to the end of the roll, either turn around or tandem walk backward.

| _____ Reps _____ Sets _____ X Day _____ Hold | _____ Reps _____ Sets _____ X Day _____ Hold |
|---|---|
| **83** Notes: | **84** Notes: |

SINGLE LEG STANCE - ABDUCTION

Place a half foam roll on the ground in a side-to-side direction. Balance on one leg and move the opposite leg to the side.

SINGLE LEG STANCE - ABDUCTION

Place a half foam roll on the ground in a forward-back direction. Balance on one leg with the opposite leg to the side.

| _____ Reps _____ Sets _____ X Day _____ Hold | _____ Reps _____ Sets _____ X Day _____ Hold |
|---|---|
| **85** Notes: | **86** Notes: |

SINGLE LEG STANCE – FORWARD KICK

Place a half foam roll on the ground in a forward-back direction. Balance on one leg and move the opposite leg forward.

SINGLE LEG STANCE – HAMSTRING CURL

Place a half foam roll on the ground in a forward-back direction. Balance on one leg and with the opposite leg, bend the knee backwards as shown.

| _____ Reps _____ Sets _____ X Day _____ Hold | | _____ Reps _____ Sets _____ X Day _____ Hold |
|---|---|---|
| **87** | Notes: | **88** | Notes: |

**SINGLE LEG SQUAT – LEG FORWARD**

Place a half foam roll on the ground in a forward-back direction. Balance on one leg with a slight bend in the supporting knee and move the opposite leg forward. Straighten supporting knee and repeat.

**SINGLE LEG SQUAT – LEG BACKWARDS**

Place a half foam roll on the ground in a forward-back direction. Balance on one leg with a slight bend in the supporting knee and with the opposite leg, move the leg backwards as shown with bent knee. Straighten supporting knee and repeat.

## STAIR STEP – *To progress, increase step height*

| _____ Reps _____ Sets _____ X Day _____ Hold | | _____ Reps _____ Sets _____ X Day _____ Hold |
|---|---|---|
| **89** | Notes: | **90** | Notes: |

**TOE TAP OR HEEL PLACEMENT**

While standing with both feet on the floor, place one foot on the top of the step. Next, return the foot back to the floor and then repeat with the other leg.
You can either put your foot up for several repetitions or alternate.

**PULL UP FOOT TOUCHES ON STEP**

Whie standing with both feet on the ground, put one foot on the step. Push through the foot straightening the knee until the opposite foot is off the ground. Lower the foot back to the starting position. Repeat with the opposite foot for several repetitions.

| | _____ Reps _____ Sets _____X Day _____Hold |
|---|---|
| **91** | **Notes:** |

ALTERNATING SUSTAINED FOOT TOUCHES ON STEP

Whie standing with both feet on the ground,  put one foot on the step. Push through the foot straightening the knee until the opposite foot is also on the step.  Step off backwards to the starting position.  Repeat with the opposite foot for several repetitions.

| | _____ Reps _____ Sets _____X Day _____Hold |
|---|---|
| **92** | **Notes:** |

STEP UP AND OVER

Step up onto the step and then onto the ground on the other side.  Turn around and repeat.
Repeat  several repetitions on one side and then the other or alternate legs.

| | _____ Reps _____ Sets _____X Day _____Hold |
|---|---|
| **93** | **Notes:** |

FORWARD SWING THROUGH STEP

Step up onto the step without stopping on the top, swing opposite leg through and onto the floor on the other side.

| | _____ Reps _____ Sets _____X Day _____Hold |
|---|---|
| **94** | **Notes:** |

SIDE STEPPING

******REPEAT STEPS 89-93 from a side approach****

**Agility**

| EXERCISE<br>Agility/Reactivity/Speed | EXERCISE NUMBER | NOTES |
|---|---|---|
| Four Square Drills | 1 | |
| Dots | 2 | |
| Ladder Drills | 3 | |
| Box Drills | 4 | |
| Cones | 5 | |
| Hurdles | 6 | |

# Agility/Reactivity/Speed

According to the Twist Conditioning workbook, "Agility is the ability to link several fundamental movement skills into a multidirectional pattern. Reaction skills are the 'whole body' responsiveness to external stimuli, as well as muscle and joint internal reactivity. Quickness is the ability to explosively initiate movement from a stationary position, as well as shifting the gears of speed". (*Twist, Peter, Twist Agility, Quickness and & Reactivity Workbook, 2009, pg 16*)

Agility is a combination of acceleration, deceleration, coordination, power, strength and dynamic balance. With agility training, always keep your head in a neutral position looking straight ahead no matter which way you turn. "Powerful arm movement during transitional and directional changes is essential in order to reacquire a high rate of speed". (*Brown & Ferrigno, 2005, pp 73-74*)

Agility exercises can be done with cones, hurdles, dots or squares on the floor, box drills, Bosu or ladders. Agility can also be high impact or explosive movements. If you are not comfortable with this in the beginning or have any contraindications, stick with low impact movements. In other words, if you are jumping over hurdles, keep them low to the ground and jump over with one leg leading for low impact and jump with both legs for high impact.

If you are doing box drills or Bosu, please do NOT JUMP off backwards.

## AGILITY / SPEED / REACTIVITY

### 4 Square Drills

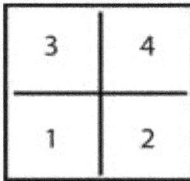 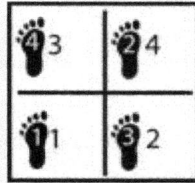 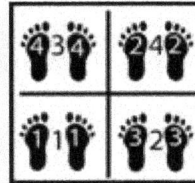 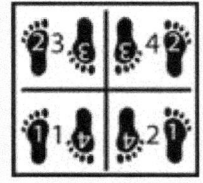

### Dots

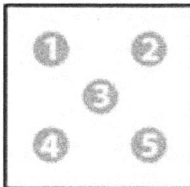 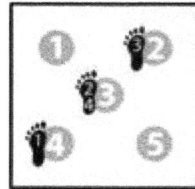 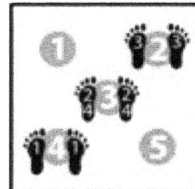 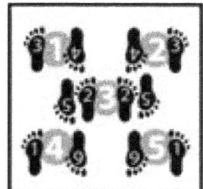

### Ladder

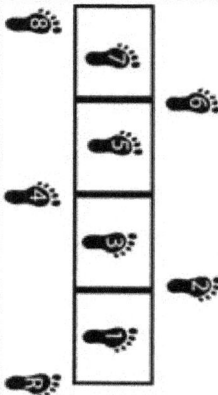 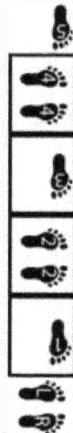 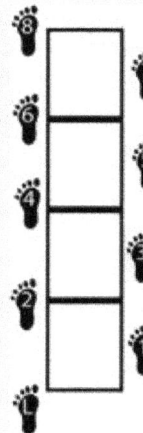 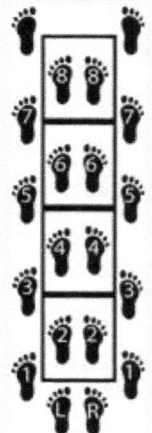

**Box Drills** – Box should be no higher than the middle of your shin.  This can be done on Bosu for balance.

| | | | |
|---|---|---|---|
| Alt Tap Box With Foot | Down Up Both Feet Together | Quickly Move Side to Side | Down Up Both Feet Together |

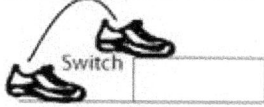

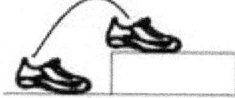

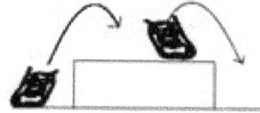

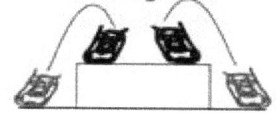

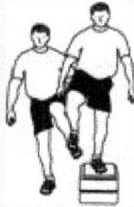

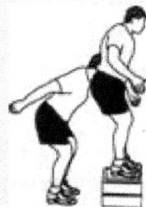

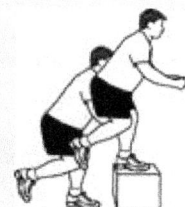

**Cones**

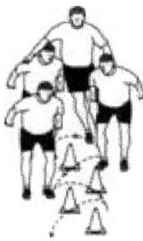

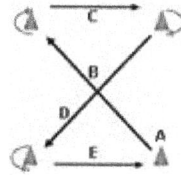

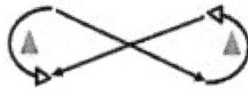

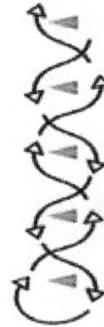

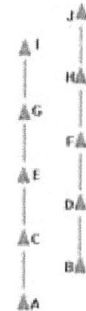

**Hurdles** – can run or jump over hurdles

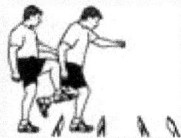

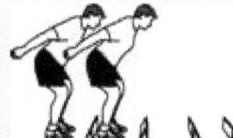

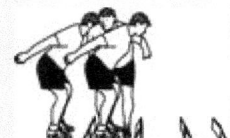

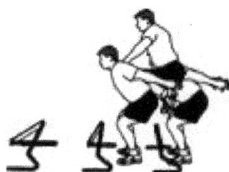

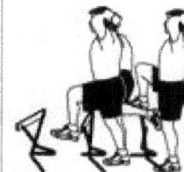

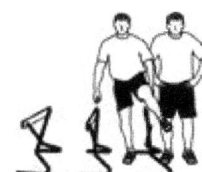

# Endurance / Aerobic Capacity

## Aerobic - with oxygen: Muscular and Cardiovascular

Many repetitions with sub-maximal weight (weight that is less than the maximum you can lift).

Muscular endurance is the ability of the muscle or group of muscles to sustain repeated contractions against resistance for an extended period of time. This is needed to build muscle. (See *Strengthening*). Cardiovascular endurance is the ability of the heart, lungs and blood vessels to deliver oxygen to working muscles and tissues, as well as the ability of those muscles and tissues to utilize that oxygen. This is needed to help endure long runs or sustained activity, as with biking or running. In short, endurance or aerobic exercises increase the heart rate and respiratory rate.

As far as long-term performance goes, there are two types of muscle fibers that can determine the likelihood of success: slow and fast twitch, which may determine whether you are more likely to be a power-lifter or sprinter (*fast twitch*), or a marathon runner (*slow twitch*). Your ability depends on the distribution of these fibers in the body. In other words, you could have a certain percentage of slow twitch in your biceps, but a different percentage in your quadriceps. There is some controversy over whether you can change the percentage or distribution of these fibers with endurance training or training for a specific event, although you may be able to change the glycolytic capacity.

| | |
|---|---|
| **Type of Fibers** | *Slow twitch fibers:* Have a high aerobic capacity and are resistant to fatigue. People that have a higher percentage of slow twitch fibers tend to have better endurance abilities.<br><br>*Fast twitch fibers:* Contract faster than slow twitch, and thus fatigue faster. People that have a higher percentage of fast twitch fibers tend to have better sprinting or muscle building abilities. |

The following research is from the: **MAYO CLINIC**

Mayo Clinic - *https://www.mayoclinic.org/healthy-lifestyle/fitness/in-depth/aerobic-exercise/art-20045541*

Regular aerobic activity, such as walking, bicycling or swimming, can help you live longer and healthier. Need motivation? See how aerobic exercise affects your heart, lungs and blood flow.

### How your body responds to aerobic exercise

During aerobic activity, you repeatedly move large muscles in your arms, legs and hips. You'll notice your body's responses quickly.

You'll breathe faster and more deeply. This maximizes the amount of oxygen in your blood. Your heart will beat faster, which increases blood flow to your muscles and back to your lungs.

Your small blood vessels (capillaries) will widen to deliver more oxygen to your muscles and carry away waste products, such as carbon dioxide and lactic acid.

Your body will even release endorphins, natural painkillers that promote an increased sense of well-being.

### What aerobic exercise does for your health.

Regardless of age, weight or athletic ability, aerobic activity is good for you. As your body adapts to regular aerobic exercise, you will get stronger and fitter.

Consider the following 10 ways that aerobic activity can help you feel better and enjoy life to the fullest on the next page.

## Aerobic activity can help you:

1. **Keep excess pounds at bay**
   Combined with a healthy diet, aerobic exercise helps you lose weight and keep it off.

2. **Increase your stamina**
   You may feel tired when you first start regular aerobic exercise. But over the long term, you'll enjoy increased stamina and reduced fatigue.

3. **Ward off viral illnesses**
   Aerobic exercise activates your immune system in a good way. This may leave you less susceptible to minor viral illnesses, such as colds and flu.

4. **Reduce your health risks**
   Aerobic exercise reduces the risk of many conditions, including obesity, heart disease, high blood pressure, type 2 diabetes, metabolic syndrome, stroke and certain types of cancer.

   Weight-bearing aerobic exercises, such as walking, help decrease the risk of osteoporosis.

5. **Manage chronic conditions**
   Aerobic exercise may help lower blood pressure and control blood sugar. If you have coronary artery disease, aerobic exercise may help you manage your condition.

6. **Strengthen your heart**
   A stronger heart doesn't need to beat as fast. A stronger heart also pumps blood more efficiently, which improves blood flow to all parts of your body.

7. **Keep your arteries clear**
   Aerobic exercise boosts your high-density lipoprotein (HDL), the "good," cholesterol, and lowers your low-density lipoprotein (LDL), the "bad," cholesterol. This may result in less buildup of plaques in your arteries.

8. **Boost your mood**
   Aerobic exercise may ease the gloominess of depression, reduce the tension associated with anxiety and promote relaxation.

9. **Stay active and independent as you age**
   Aerobic exercise keeps your muscles strong, which can help you maintain mobility as you get older. Studies have found that regular physical activity may help protect memory, reasoning, judgment and thinking skills (cognitive function) in older adults and may improve cognitive function in young adults.

10. **Live longer**
    Studies show that people who participate in regular aerobic exercise live longer than those who don't exercise regularly.

## Take the first step

Ready to get more active? Great. Just remember to start with small steps. If you've been inactive for a long time or if you have a chronic health condition, get your doctor's OK before you start. When you're ready to begin exercising, start slowly. You might walk five minutes in the morning and five minutes in the evening.
The next day, add a few minutes to each walking session. Pick up the pace a bit, too. Soon, you could be walking briskly for at least 30 minutes a day and reaping all the benefits of regular aerobic activity.

Other options for aerobic exercise could include cross-country skiing, aerobic dancing, swimming, stair climbing, bicycling, jogging, elliptical training or rowing.

(Mayo Clinic - *https://www.mayoclinic.org/healthy-lifestyle/fitness/in-depth/aerobic-exercise/art-20045541*)

# Calories

Calorie: A unit of food energy. The word calorie is ordinarily used instead of the more precise, scientific term kilocalorie. A kilocalorie represents the amount of energy required to raise the temperature of a liter of water 1' centigrade at sea level. Technically, a kilocalorie represents 1,000 true calories of energy. *(MedicineNet.com)*

Calories are a measurement tool, like inches or cups. Calories measure the energy a food or beverage provides from the carbohydrate, fat, protein, and alcohol* it contains. Calories give you the fuel or energy you need to work and play – even to rest and sleep! When choosing what to eat and drink, it's important to get the right mix – enough nutrients without too many calories. Paying attention to calories is an important part of managing your weight. The amount of calories you need are different if you want to gain, lose, or maintain your weight. Tracking what and how much you eat, and drink can help you better understand your calorie intake over time. Each person's body may have different needs for calories and exercise. A healthy lifestyle requires balance in the foods you eat, the beverages you drink, the way you do daily activities, adequate sleep, stress management, and in the amount of activity in your daily routine. (*ChooseMyPlate.gov & CDC*)

**Example of Activities and Calories Burned** (*ChooseMyPlate.gov*)
A 154-pound man who is 5' 10" will use up (burn) about the number of calories listed doing each activity below. Those who weigh more will use more calories; those who weigh less will use fewer calories. The calorie values listed include both calories used by the activity and the calories used for normal body functioning during the activity time.

| EXAMPLE | Approximate calories used (burned) by a 154-pound man | |
|---|---|---|
| **MODERATE** physical activities: | In 1 hour | In 30 minutes |
| Hiking | 370 | 185 |
| Light gardening/ yard work | 330 | 165 |
| Dancing | 330 | 165 |
| Golf (walking and carrying clubs) | 330 | 165 |
| Bicycling (less than 10 mph) | 290 | 145 |
| Walking (3.5 mph) | 280 | 140 |
| Weight training (general light workout) | 220 | 110 |
| Stretching | 180 | 90 |
| **VIGOROUS** physical activities: | In 1 hour | In 30 minutes |
| Running/ jogging (5 mph) | 590 | 295 |
| Bicycling (more than 10 mph) | 590 | 295 |
| Swimming (slow freestyle laps) | 510 | 255 |
| Aerobics | 480 | 240 |
| Walking (4.5 mph) | 460 | 230 |
| Heavy yard work (chopping wood) | 440 | 220 |
| Weightlifting (vigorous effort) | 440 | 220 |
| Basketball (vigorous) | 440 | 220 |

# References

### *Also, Some Good Books, Websites & DVD'*

ACE Idea Fitness Journal: *Martina M. Cartwright, PhD, RD http://www.ideafit.com/fitness-library/protein-today-are-consumers-getting-too-much-of-a-good-thing?ACE_ACCESS=ebec6bcf61abff08f7b1d8b27c555758*

ACE Senior Fitness Manual, *American Council on Exercise* (2014)

American Physical Therapy Association, (APTA), 2007. *Basic Science for Animal Physical Therapy: Canine, 2nd edition*

Arleigh J Reynolds, DVM, PhD - *www.absasleddogracing.org.uk/newgang/src/gangline/role.htm*

Australian Institute of Sports - *http://www.ausport.gov.au*

*BodyBuilder.com*

Brown & Ferrigno, (2005). *Training for Speed, Agility and Quickness*, Champaign, IL: Human Kinetics.

Bryant, C & Green, D, editors (2003), *Ace Personal Trainer Manual, 3rd ed.*, San Diego, CA: American Council on Exercise (ACE)

*ChooseMyPlate.gov*

*Examine.com*

*ExRx.net*

Feher & Szunyoghy (1996). *Cyclopedia Anatomicae,* Tess Press

Gillette, R (2002). Temperature Regulation of the Dog. Retrieved June 2011 from *http://www.sportsvet.com/11Nwsltr.PDF*

Gillette, R (2008). *Feeding the Canine Athlete for Optimal Performance.* Retrieved September 25, 2008 from *www.sports vet.com/Art3.html.*

Glucose (Wikipedia) - *http://en.wikipedia.org/wiki/Glucose*

Glycemic Index (Wikipedia) - *http://en.wikipedia.org/wiki/Glycemic_index*

*LiveStrong.com*

Mayo Clinic - *https://www.mayoclinic.org/healthy-lifestyle/fitness/in-depth/aerobic-exercise/art-20045541*

*MedicineNet.com*

Myofascial Release: ( Wikipedia) - https://en.wikipedia.org/wiki/Myofascial_release

Rikli, Roberta and Jones, Jessie (2013) *Senior Fitness Test Manual, 2nd Ed.,*

Strength Training: (Wikipedia) *http://en.wikipedia.org/wiki/Strength_training*

Twist, Peter (2009). *Twist Agility, Quickness and & Reactivity Workbook.* British Columbia: Twist Conditioning, Inc. University of Maryland Medical Center.com

*Workout Australia*

# Thank You to:

## My Husband
*Model*
For his support through my battle with cancer and while writing this and previous books.
Also, for the patience and hours he put in modeling for this book.

## My Daughter
For giving me artistic inspiration and providing artwork for my previous books.

## My Grandchildren
## Just Because

## God
For giving me the strength to overcome cancer and the wisdom to write these books.

# Certifications, Continuing Education and License

**Physical Therapist Assistant – L/PTA – 30 years in both Home Therapy and Short-Term Rehab facilities**

**ACE Certified Personal Trainer – CPT**
- o **Functional Training Specialist**
- o **Therapeutic Exercise Specialist**
- o **Senior Fitness Specialist**
- o **Nutrition and Fitness Specialist**

**©Klose Education**
- o **Certified Lymphedema Therapist – CLT**
- o **Strength After Breast Cancer – Strength ABC**
- o **Breast Cancer Rehabilitation**

**©Cancer Exercise Specialist Institute – CETI**
- o **Cancer Exercise Specialist – CES**
- o **Breast Cancer Recovery BOSU(R) Specialist Advanced Qualification**
- o **Pilates Mat Certificate**

**©MedFit**
- o **Medical Fitness Specialist**
- o **Parkinson's Disease Fitness Specialist**
- o **Arthritis Fitness Specialist**

**©Pink Ribbon Program**

**©The BioMechanics Method - Corrective Exercise Specialist**

**©ISSA - DNA-Based Fitness Coach**

www.ingramcontent.com/pod-product-compliance
Lightning Source LLC
Chambersburg PA
CBHW052110020426
42335CB00021B/2697